The Complete Guide to Vegetarian and Pescatarian Keto Diet

Know and Choose the Perfect Diet for You

Maya Bryce

© **Copyright 2020 - All rights reserved.**

The content contained within this book may not be reproduced, duplicated or transmitted without direct written permission from the author or the publisher.

Under no circumstances will any blame or legal responsibility be held against the publisher, or author, for any damages, reparation, or monetary loss due to the information contained within this book, either directly or indirectly.

Legal Notice:

This book is copyright protected. It is only for personal use. You cannot amend, distribute, sell, use, quote or paraphrase any part, or the content within this book, without the consent of the author or publisher.

Disclaimer Notice:

Please note the information contained within this document is for educational and entertainment purposes only. All effort has been executed to present accurate, up to date, reliable, complete information. No warranties of any kind are declared or implied.

Readers acknowledge that the author is not engaged in the rendering of legal, financial, medical or professional advice. The content within this book has been derived from various sources. Please consult a licensed professional before attempting any techniques outlined in this book.

By reading this document, the reader agrees that under no circumstances is the author responsible for any losses, direct or indirect, that are incurred as a result of the use of the information contained within this document, including, but not limited to, errors, omissions, or inaccuracies.

Table of Contents

Table of Contents..5
Introduction to Vegetarian Keto Diet........................14
    The Vegetarian Keto Diet Plan..............................17
Chapter 1: The Keto Diet &..19
the Vegetarian Diet..19
    The Ketogenic Diet...20
        The History of the Ketogenic Diet.....................24
        The Advantages of the Ketogenic Diet...............25
        The Disadvantages of the Ketogenic Diet..........26
    The Vegetarian Diet..29
        The History of the Vegetarian Diet....................31
        The Advantages of the Vegetarian Diet.............32
        The Disadvantages of the Vegetarian Diet........33
    The Bottom Line...34
Chapter 2: How to Get Started on the Vegetarian Keto Diet 37

Myths of the Ketogenic Diet..................................39

Steps to the Ketogenic Diet....................................44

Burning Unwanted Fat..53

The Bottom Line...56

Chapter 3: Vegetarian Keto Foods............................59

The Forbidden Foods for a Vegetarian Keto Diet..61

The Allowed Foods on the Vegetarian Keto Diet...62

The Weekly Grocery List......................................63

   Beverages..63

   Fruits...64

   Vegetables...64

   The Fridge & Freezer Staples............................65

   Pantry Staples..66

   Nuts & Seeds..66

   Herbs & Spices...67

   Nut & Seed Butters..67

   Healthy Oils...68

   Sauces & Condiments.....................................68

Sweeteners..68

The Bottom Line...69

Chapter 4: Keto-Friendly Fruits & Vegetables 71

Keto-Friendly Fruits..71

Keto-Friendly Vegetables..78

Keto-Friendly Veggie & Fruit Recipes...................86

    Keto Chocolate Ice Cream................................86

    Berry Pops..88

    Tomato Soup...91

    Roasted Broccoli..93

    Low-Carb Cauliflower Hash Browns.................95

    Creamy Spinach...97

The Bottom Line...99

Chapter 5: Vegetarian Keto Diet Breakfast Ideas.....101

Blueberry Pancakes..101

Low-Carb Brownie Muffins.....................................104

Veggie Scramble...106

Keto Breakfast Granola...108

Mixed Berry Smoothie..110

Low-Carb Oatmeal...112

Chapter 6: Vegetarian Keto Diet Lunch Ideas..........114

Collard Green Veggie Wraps...................................114

Red Pepper Spinach Salad.......................................117

Keto Club Salad...118

Grilled Cheese Zucchini 121

Asparagus Fries 124

Avocado Taco..127

Mushroom & Avocado Salad..................................130

Chapter 7: Vegetarian Keto Diet Dinner Ideas.........133

Keto Broccoli Salad..133

Zucchini Skins..135

Tofu & Bok Choy..137

Grilled Eggplant...141

Caprese Salad...143

Broccoli Creamy Casserole.....................................145

Cauliflower Broccoli Stir Fry..................................148

Chapter 8: Vegetarian Keto Diet Snack Ideas 152

    Keto Cucumber Sushi..152

    Avocado 'Potato' Chip..154

    Strawberry Milkshake..155

    Mixed Berries Fruit Roll Ups..................................157

    Low Carb Pumpkin Spice Fat Bombs...................160

    Portobello Mushroom Fries....................................162

    Avocado & Goat Cheese Bites................................165

Chapter 9: Vegetarian Keto Dessert Ideas................168

    Blackberry Pudding...168

    Coconut Chip Cookies 170

    Peanut Butter Balls..173

    Frosty...174

    Low-Carb Carrot Cake 176

    Low-Carb Chia Pudding...179

    Peanut Butter Chocolate Cups 181

Conclusion...185

Introduction to Pescatarian Keto Diet.......................187

Chapter 1: The Basics of the Keto Diet....................193

    What Is Keto?...193

    What Are the Benefits of Keto?...........................195

Chapter 2: Why Choose the Keto Lifestyle?............201

    Weight Loss..201

    Lower Your Cholesterol..................................203

    Reduce Aging..204

Chapter 3: Who is a Pescatarian?..........................210

    What do Pescatarians Eat?..............................211

    What Did a Pescatarian Eat?...........................212

    What Doesn't a Pescatarian Eat?....................213

    Reasons to Change Your Lifestyle...................214

    Reasons to Follow a Pescatarian Diet..............215

    The Health Benefits of a Pescatarian Lifestyle.....217

    Benefits of Adding Fish to a Diet......................218

Chapter 4: The Pescatarian Diet............................221

Chapter 5: Preparing your Pescatarian Kitchen......227

    Smart Spending..233

Selecting and Preparing Fish And Seafood.........235

Chapter 6: Prepping for The Ketogenic Diet............237

Chapter 7: Mistakes to Avoid on A Ketogenic Diet..244

Mistake #1: Bad Mindset......................................244

Mistake #2: Eating Too Much.............................245

Mistake #3: Not Testing..246

Mistake #4: Not Eating Enough Nutrient-Dense Foods..247

Mistake #5: Eating Toxic, Inflammatory Foods - Even if They're Low Carb...249

Mistake #6: Ignoring Sleep, Exercise, and Stress 251

Mistake #7: Not Being Patient.............................251

Mistake #8: Not Eating Enough Fiber.................252

Chapter 8: Weight Loss and Exercise 253

Chapter 9: Strict Diet for Fat Burning.....................261

Eat More Cruciferous Vegetables.........................261

How to Do It:..266

Chapter 10: Reaching Your Goal..........................271

Chapter 11: Advantages and Disadvantages of Ketogenic Diet..276

Advantages of Keto Diet..................................276

Disadvantages of Keto Diet.............................281

Chapter 12: The Best Ways to Lose Weight Fast.....283

Eat Out Less 283

Don't Skip Meals 285

Eat Less at Night 286

Sleep 287

Team Up 287

Mindful Eating 289

Chapter 13: Weight Loss Affirmations 291

Chapter 14: 10 Tasty And Healthy Recipes............298

Salmon Skewers..298

Coconut Salmon with Napa Cabbage..................299

Keto Tuna Casserole.....................................302

Baked Fish Fillets with Vegetables in Foil...........304

Baked Salmon with Almonds and Cream Sauce. 306

Spring Greens Soup......................................308

Celery Soup...309

Eggplant Stew...311

Asparagus Frittata..313

Bell Peppers Soup...314

Chapter 15: Top Tips and Cautions to Stay Pescatarian 317

Get Your Carbs From Vegetables........................317

Get Plenty Of Sleep 319

Lower Your Stress 319

Increase Your Salt Intake 320

Engage In Physical Activity 321

Keep Track Of Your Carb Macronutrients...........322

Clean Your Kitchen 323

Have Quick Meals Ready 324

Be Mindful When Eating Out 325

Try Meal Prepping 326

Conclusion...327

Introduction to Vegetarian Keto Diet

The vegetarian ketogenic diet changed my life.

This is a statement you might have heard before, but honestly, the introduction of both of these eating styles turned my eating habits around for the better, and better yet, they have aided me in losing the unwanted weight, which had been with me since childhood.

As someone who has struggled with weight loss most of my life, the constantly inflating belly, jiggling arms, and jean-ruining rubbing thighs are hauntingly familiar to me. Another familiar struggle is accepting that second offer of cake, consuming the extra slice of pizza because no one else will, and standing in the candy aisle at grocery stores deciding between a chocolate bar or leaving the aisle to buy some household goods that are actually needed at home.

The above-mentioned struggles and many others were part of my life for a long time until shrugging and laughing about my weight could no longer hide the fact that there was seriously something wrong with my eating habits.

Two of the first things that needed to change though were my thoughts and beliefs around weight loss and healthy eating. There were some fallacious ideas about myself that were constantly swimming around my head, which were often the cause of me not being able to fully commit to or complete a diet. My biggest misconception was believing there was a quick and easy way to lose weight. Although, it did finally dawn on me that there was no quick and easy fix to shedding those extra pounds.

Another one of my deterring thoughts was believing there was nothing wrong with my weight or eating habits. However, my constant discomfort with my body and the fact that my after three months new clothes got too tight clearly showed me that was not the truth. There was also the most backward and humiliating thought of all: physical exercise was merely a suggestion. Nonetheless, it soon became clear to me that physical exercise was one of the best ways to burn more calories than you consumed.

The vegetarian lifestyle had been part of my life for years before my weight became an issue and the ketogenic diet came onto the scene. Becoming a vegetarian was an eating style that came with new friends in my life who were either vegetarians or vegans. They did not force their lifestyle on me or trash-talk meat, but it was one of those 'show me your friends and I will show you your future' sort of scenarios. Although, I did not commit to the diet until some research and some eye-opening documentaries were undertaken, which taught me that meat wasn't the 'big cheese' everyone made it out to be. After that, it was easy to commit to the diet and meat was not a food that I missed in my life. However, there was more weight gain than loss because to substitute for the lack of meat and filling meals, my intake of vegetarian/vegan-friendly carbs and sugars increased.

Eventually though, the effect these carbs and sugars had become evident and cutting down my intake and going for 45-minute walks seemed like the solution; however, it wasn't until the ketogenic diet that everything really began to change.

As a vegetarian, you already practice watching what you eat but that is only with meat or some dairy products; the ketogenic diet is on another level, and the combination of both of these diets results in you eating healthier and less.

Nevertheless, once my combination of both of these eating styles began, there was no turning back. Another great thing was that working out became a regular routine in my life; the 45 minutes walks turned to intense cardio workouts that my body truly enjoyed. Eventually, as the weeks and months went by, my clothes became loose and baggy, the flat stomach I woke up to in the mornings remained intact even after breakfast, lunch, and dinner, and everything stayed where it is supposed to and these are the results that have kept me eating healthy and maintaining my new figure.

The Vegetarian Keto Diet Plan

Every person is different and one way does not always suit everyone, which is why the *Vegetarian Keto Diet Plan: How to Lose Weight Eating Healthy and Tasty Food* was written as a guide for all vegetarians seeking to implement the effects of the ketogenic diet into their lives.

If you've been looking for information about how to incorporate keto into you vegetarian lifestyle (or perhaps you want to make a complete switch to both keto and vegetarianism), then look no further as you will learn all about:

- What are the vegetarian and keto diets with the pros and cons to following this lifestyle
- Myths related to keto so you know what you are in for and what to expect

- Steps to follow to get you started on this new journey

- How to lose weight on the vegetarian keto diet

- Vegetarian keto-friendly foods you may eat (as well as the foods to avoid)

Tasty recipes you and your family can enjoy!

We want you to have a clear understanding about the vegetarian keto diet, attain progressive beliefs and thoughts that will only launch you upward and forward in your weight loss journey, and the ability to confidently state you know exactly what to do to lose weight, eating healthy vegetarian food the keto way.

Chapter 1: The Keto Diet &

the Vegetarian Diet

The vegetarian keto diet is a combination of the ketogenic diet and the vegetarian diet. There is still some debate around the effects of the ketogenic diet but the same debate usually takes place around the vegetarian diet, and many of you reading this guide will be very aware there will always be someone saying something discouraging about eating styles that require you to cut out what the rest of the population considers to be 'essential' foods.

At the end of the day, if a life with a minuscule amount of carbs is something you can commit to, then you can make the ketogenic diet a permanent diet in your life. However, if you cannot bear to be without carbs, then we recommend you only use the ketogenic diet for three to maybe six months before returning to an everyday vegetarian diet. We will now be discussing the vegetarian and ketogenic diet at their core so we can better understand how these two diets can work together.

The Ketogenic Diet

The everyday diet consists of macronutrients.

And macronutrients or macros are our sources of nutrients; they are what we count when calculating calories and these macros are carbohydrates, fat, and protein. The recommended diet the majority of us grew up on consists of a high carb intake, a moderate intake of protein, and very low fat intake, and this is the diet that best meets our nutritional needs. However, most people's diets consist of a high fat, high carb, and even high protein intake, which is due to the fact that a lot of people can't afford to eat healthier, don't have the time to eat healthier, or they eat whatever because at least they ate something.

The ketogenic diet is good at halting this kind of unhealthy eating because on keto you are encouraged to consume more fats, moderate protein, and much fewer carbs. However, the suggested fats you should consume on the ketogenic diet are the good kinds of fat, good kinds of (low) carbs, and the good kinds of protein.

No sugary or starchy fats and carbs are to be found here.

What the ketogenic diet triggers is ketosis, which is a metabolic state that occurs in the body when the body is forced to burn fat for energy instead of carbohydrates. Carbohydrates are the regular fuel source for the body and glucose, which is produced by carbohydrates, is the default fuel for the brain. During ketosis, though, both the brain and body burn fat for energy, which is how you can burn fat (both the excess your body has stored and from dietary sources) and lose weight while you follow the keto diet.

When you are on the ketogenic diet, you are encouraged to consume foods, and you earn your calories through a diet that is high in fat, moderate in protein, and low in carbohydrates. Essentially, you must completely cut out all foods high in carbohydrates (grains, sugar, starch, etc.) from your diet, and invite good fats (avocados, olive oil, non-starchy vegetables, etc.) into your diet.

There are eight kinds of ketogenic diets. The standard ketogenic diet is the most common and is the basis for most, if not all, the other kinds of keto diets people follow.

#1. Standard Ketogenic Diet (SKD)

As the most common type of ketogenic diet, you can consume up to 20 to 50 grams of carbohydrates, 40 to 60 grams of protein, and 165 grams of fat. However, there is no set limit for fat because most of our calories should come from our fat intake so take the fat intake here as a suggestion.

#2. Very-Low-Carb Ketogenic Diet (VLCKD)

The very-low-carb ketogenic refers to a standard ketogenic diet but the diet consists of lower carb intake. On this diet, many people restrict their daily intake of carbs to between 20 and 30 grams.

#3. Well-Formulated Ketogenic Diet (WFKD)

The diet is similar to the *standard ketogenic diet* but in this instance, the macronutrients of fat, protein, and carbohydrates are identical to the ratios of the standard ketogenic diet. With this form of keto, there is a higher chance of ketosis taking place in the body. With WFKD you have to stick to the set and recommended amounts of fat (165 grams), protein (40 grams), and carbs (20 grams). There is a set limit to fat.

#4. MCT Ketogenic Diet

The MCT ketogenic diet is based on the SKD, but the diet uses MCT oils to create 60% of the fats that will be burnt by the body. MCTs create more ketones per ounce of fat than the long-chain triglycerides, which are found in the standard everyday diet. Using MCT oils in your ketogenic diet ensures you will maintain ketosis and, at the same time, be able to eat more carbohydrates and protein. Consuming too much

MCTs, especially on an inconsistent and unbalanced diet, can result in an upset stomach.

#5. Calorie-Restricted Ketogenic Diet

The calorie-restricted ketogenic diet restricts calories to a set amount. For women, 2,000 calories are the recommended maximum number of calories, and the recommended maximum calorie intake for men is 2,500. However, this keto diet could restrict your calorie intake to the minimum amount which is 1,200 calories.

#6. Cyclical Ketogenic Diet (CKD)

Another name for the cyclical ketogenic diet is the carb back-loading diet.

This is the keto diet that is recommended for athletes. Naturally, the diet allows athletes to enjoy a higher concentration of carbohydrates two days out of the week, which allows them to regain the glycogen in their muscles that was lost because of their intense training and working out schedules.

#7. Targeted Ketogenic Diet (TKD)

A combination of the standard ketogenic diet and the cyclical ketogenic diet is what the targeted ketogenic diet consists of. Basically, the diet allows you to consume more carbohydrates, but only on the days you exercise.

#8. High-Protein Ketogenic Diet

The high-protein ketogenic diet was created to assist individuals who need to lose weight for health reasons. The diet is based on the standard ketogenic diet and the diet consists of 35% protein, 60% fat, and 5% carbs.

The History of the Ketogenic Diet

Back in the 1920s and 1930s, the ketogenic diet was created and used to treat adults and children with epilepsy. Although, it is said the diet was temporarily abandoned when anticonvulsant therapies were introduced. On the other hand, the new medications failed to achieve the same astounding results as the ketogenic diet—especially in children, and so the ketogenic diet was reintroduced shortly after this assessment was made.

It seems that three individuals partook in the discovery of the keto diet.

Rollin Woodyatt was the endocrinologist who discovered that three kinds of ketone bodies—acetone, beta-hydroxybutyrate, and acetoacetate—were generated in the liver as a result of starvation or a high in fat and low in carb diet.

However, it was Russel Wilder of the Mayo Clinic who named the above-mentioned reaction in the body, discovered by Woodyatt, the ketogenic diet. And it was Peter Huttenlocher who first altered the keto diet so patients on the treatment could consume more protein and carbohydrates. Huttenlocher was able to make this alternation by suggesting that 60% of his patients' fat intake be gained mostly from MCT oils.

The Advantages of the Ketogenic Diet

#1. Weight Loss

With the ketogenic diet, the body enters a state of ketosis, and as a result, more ketones are created in the body. The ketones become the main source of energy for both the body and the brain. Usually, the brain burns the glucose from carbohydrates for energy and the body burns carbohydrates for energy. However, on the keto diet, the body and the brain burn fat for energy, so no excess fat is stored, and that results in weight loss.

#2. Epilepsy

As we have mentioned, the ketogenic was created as a therapeutic treatment for children and adults with epilepsy. The treatment was shortly abandoned but reintroduced to treat children who experienced epileptic seizures.

#3. Type 2 Diabetes

The low carb requirement of the ketogenic diet strongly impacts glucose concentrations, and it tends to lower glucose over time. Although, if you are a type 2 diabetic, we suggest that you consult with your doctor first before using the ketogenic diet as a solution.

#4. Cancer

There are not a lot of studies in regard to the advantages keto has on cancer, but according to Satterthwaite (2018, p. 134):

> The Warburg effect has established that tumour cells can break down glucose much faster (specifically 200x faster) compared to typical cells. The theory is that by 'starving' tumour cells of glucose, you can inhibit their growth and help prevent cancer.

The Disadvantages of the Ketogenic Diet

#1. Keto Flu

The symptoms of the keto flu are constipation, fatigue, 'foggy brain', headaches, hunger, and irritability. The keto flu usually occurs at the start of the ketogenic diet (during the first week or two), and is due to the change in your diet; that is, cutting carbohydrates from your diet. Our suggestion is you remain well-rested and hydrated during the course of the diet to avoid and minimize your symptoms. Although, it is possible to avoid the keto flu by taking things slowly, as in changing your diet little by little instead of all at once.

#2. **Nutrient Deficiencies**

Nutrients are essential in any diet and for the body to function the way it should. We suggest that you follow the directions in this guide and only make alterations when you are certain you will not be cutting any needed nutrients out of your diet.

#3. **Gut Health**

Due to the lack of fiber and certain fruits in the keto diet, you might have issues in terms of being regular. There are other keto-friendly foods that offer you the needed amount of fiber, but we suggest you also remember to drink water along with following a balanced diet.

#4. **Obedience**

Maintaining any diet takes commitment, and dieting is occasionally easier said than done. With this diet, you will need to remain focused as not to self-sabotage by consuming the incorrect foods or giving up. We suggest you commit what is required of you to heart, remember the reason why you are doing this, and adhere to the guidelines written in this guide to assist you.

The Vegetarian Diet

The vegetarian diet—vegetarianism—is a diet that is meat, fish, and fowl flesh free. Mostly, we know vegetarians as environmentalists and individuals who are active in the fight regarding animal cruelty. There are only a few vegetarians—when asked— who are vegetarians purely for the health benefits.

Vegetarianism consists of about seven categories, but there are three kinds of vegetarian diets that are not considered to be "true" vegetarian.

Not True Vegetarian Diets

#1. Pescatarian

Pescatarians are individuals who occasionally consume fish and other seafoods but they do not consume any other animal flesh and some do not even consume animal by-products.

#2. Pollotarian

Pollotarians are people committed to the vegetarian diet but they often consume chicken and other poultry products, but they do not eat red or white meat.

#3. Flexitarian

Flexitarians live on a mostly plant-based diet but they occasionally consume meat, although they try to limit their meat intake when they can.

True Vegetarian Diets

On the other hand, the kinds of vegetarian diets that are considered to be the "proper" are:

#1. Veganism

Yes, veganism is a branch on the vegetarian tree.

The Vegetarian Society was first formed in England in the year 1847. However, it was only in 1944 that a man named Donald Watson coined the term vegan. He concluded that vegan would be used for vegetarians who did not consume eggs, meat, or animal by-products.

#2. Lacto Vegetarianism

Lacto vegetarians are vegetarians who do not consume any sort of animal flesh or eggs, but they use animal by-products like milk, cheese, and yogurt.

#3. Ovo Vegetarianism

The only animal by-product that ovo vegetarians consume are eggs. Ovo vegetarians do not consume red meat, white meat, fish, fowl, or any dairy products.

#4. Lacto-Ovo Vegetarianism

The most common vegetarian is a lacto-ovo vegetarian. These individuals do not consume red meat, white meat, fish, and fowl, but their veggie diet does include dairy products and eggs.

The History of the Vegetarian Diet

Historically, the vegetarian diet used to be known as the Pythagorean Diet. Yes, we are talking about the same Ancient Geek philosopher we learned about in geometry. Pythagoras was known as the father of vegetarianism for centuries, encouraging other like-minded individuals to partake in the same diet. However, in the mid-1800s, with the introduction of the Vegetarian Society in England, the Pythagorean Diet became known as the Vegetarian Diet.

Anthropologists state the vegetarian diet was popular long before Pythagoras, and they agree that the prehistoric humans' diet largely consisted of plants because plants cannot run away. Originally, the vegetarian diet was practiced for religious or ethical reasons (animal rights, etc.) However, today it is also practiced for health reasons.

The Advantages of the Vegetarian Diet

#1. Reduced Risk to Diseases

On a proper vegetarian diet, you are advised to consume whole grains, legumes, fruits, vegetables, nuts, and seeds, because these are the kinds of food packed with vitamins and minerals. The vitamins and minerals in these foods boost your health and reduce the risk of cardiovascular and gallstone disease.

#2. Prolonged Life

Certified medical practitioners have studied the link between plant-based diets and living longer, and the findings are fairly positive. Although, mindful eating, meditation and yoga, and regular exercise may play a major role in this advantage.

#3. Weight Control

It is said that plant-based diets are linked to weight loss, and that could be because we may consume less calories on a plant-based diet.

#4. Complete Nutrition

Studies have shown that it is easier to receive most of your macro and micronutrients on the vegetarian diet than on the vegan diet. Although there are some concerns regarding nutritional deficiencies on a vegetarian diet, there are more foods in the vegetarian diet that can supply you with those much-needed nutrients.

The Disadvantages of the Vegetarian Diet

#1. Nutrient Deficiencies

Vitamin B12, vitamin D, omega-3 fatty acids, calcium, and zinc are known as the vitamins that are lacking in a vegetarian diet, but sufficient nutrition can still be received through a proper and balanced vegetarian diet.

#2. Fewer Options

The vegetarian diet can be limiting at first because individuals cut out meat, seafood, and some other animal products. New vegetarians eventually learn the ropes to the vegetarian diet and their minds are opened to the healthy and tasty options and possibilities available to them.

#4. Inconvenient

The vegetarian diet can be inconvenient and time consuming with all the standing in grocery store isles reading the ingredients and checking the nutrition, minerals, and vitamins before throwing the food in your shopping cart. The same time-consuming processes can occur at restaurants and social gatherings. However, when you learn the ropes, you will become familiar with the restaurants that cater to your needs and you will be confident enough to bring your own vegetarian-friendly foods to social gatherings.

#4. Chemicals

Fruits, vegetables, and grains are often farmed using pesticides and herbicides, and the concern in the health community is that vegetarians may be more exposed to these chemicals because of their diet. The solution to this concern is to buy organic foods while the cheaper solution consists of carefully washing all the fruits and vegetables you buy and consume.

The Bottom Line

The ketogenic diet and the vegetarian diet have their differences.

Firstly, the ketogenic diet was basically created to work as a therapeutic treatment while the vegetarian diet was adopted for either religious or ethical reasons, and today the vegetarian diet seems to be more popular because of the diet's ethical background.

Secondly, the ketogenic diet focuses on limiting your intake of carbohydrates and increasing your intake of keto-friendly fats. The vegetarian diet, on the other hand, focuses on cutting or, for some vegetarians, limiting your intake of animal flesh and animal by-products.

Lastly, we can say the keto diet promotes ketosis, which is a metabolic state in the body that promotes ketones that assist you in burning fat and, thus, losing weight, while the vegetarian diet may consist of fewer calories than the regular everyday diet, which is how the vegetarian diet promotes weight loss.

There are three things these diets have in common, which is:

Firstly, the ketogenic diet and the vegetarian diet are considered to be healthy diets, and some even consider vegetarianism to be one of the healthiest diets in the world today.

Secondly, the keto diet and the vegetarian diet assist individuals in losing weight.

Lastly, the ketogenic diet and the vegetarian diet are helpful in fighting against long-term ailments such as cancer, diabetes, and cardiovascular issues.

The effects of the ketogenic and the vegetarian diets are pretty impressive. Both diets require practice and commitment, and you can really learn to be conscious about what foods you are putting in your body. Through the information in this chapter we trust you fully now understand exactly how you can learn to eat healthier and effectively lose weight on the vegetarian keto diet.

Our next chapter is packed with information about the steps you will need to take to implement the combination of these diets into your life, so we encourage you to read on, and we trust you will truly be encouraged with the next chapter.

Chapter 2: How to Get Started on the Vegetarian Keto Diet

You learned all about what the keto and vegetarian diets are in the previous chapter and may now wonder how you can combine these two. Clark (2020, p. 133) defines the vegetarian keto diet well:

> The simplest definition of the vegetarian ketogenic diet is a diet free of meat, fish, and fowl flesh that restricts carbohydrates. By eating in this way, we can reap all the benefits of the ketogenic diet while reducing our carbon footprint, decreasing animal abuse, and improving health.

Usually the biggest issues with starting a diet is the uncertainty, which could then lead you to make up excuses as to why you cannot commit fully to this diet change. When the rules are not entirely clear, we struggle to remain focused or enthusiastic about our new diet. We second-guess what we can eat, what we cannot eat, and how much we are allowed to consume during the diet all together, not to mention when something unexpected arises—how then to best deal with that and stay on your diet? And when we start to feel faint, we ask if certain activities—usually exercise—are allowed on the diet or if we are doing something wrong. Although, if you are feeling faint you might be doing something wrong or pushing too hard. Nonetheless, all the uncertainty and incorrect information leads to things like yo-yo dieting and, soon enough, we return to the 'comfortable' arms of our bad habits.

And worst of all, you gain all the weight back plus extra!

So, we recommend that you think about and even write out your intentions with this diet, and think about why you want to lose weight or eat healthier; it may sound silly, but writing things down is like talking out loud to yourself. Also write down the other diets you may have tried and why they didn't work out—more often than not the problem is in the mind. Once you write down the reason why you gave up, you can determine a path that would be solid for you. Maybe you gave up because you weren't seeing results, but everything takes time and every change consists of some struggles at the start.

Be kind and patient with yourself because you are trying something you have never tried before. We did not come walking straight out of our mother's womb, so why do we believe we can learn or develop a new habit on our first day? The first day is usually the toughest and every day after that is not always any better but eventually you will get the hang of things.

Write down your concerns, intentions, and any questions you may have, and hopefully we will answer most if not every one of your questions in this chapter.

In this chapter we look at the myths you might have heard about the ketogenic diet, tell you exactly what else you could do to lose weight on the vegetarian keto diet, and everything you need to know and consider before getting started with this lifestyle change.

Myths of the Ketogenic Diet

There are misconceptions we may have about the ketogenic diet.

Some of you may believe this is the ultimate diet to lose weight loss; however, that is not true because the reality is that the keto diet is not for everyone. There may also be some who may believe this is an unhealthy and unsafe diet—but again then people said (and still say!) the same thing about vegetarianism. If you already follow a vegetarian diet, you know it is healthy and you get all the nutrients you need The same way that there are incorrect ideas about the vegetarian diet, there is also incorrect information about the ketogenic diet. We'll look at these below so you will have the facts at hand.

#1. The Official Weight Loss Diet

Weight loss on the keto diet is possible most of all because of the person and not entirely because of the diet itself. The myth is that the ketogenic diet is the end-all-and-be-all diet, but this diet does not work for everyone because every individual does have different dietary needs.

Although, there are alterations that can be made or different variations of the diet can be tried like the different types of keto diets you learned about in our first chapter, but this diet does not always work in the same way for everyone.

The thing to do is experiment with the ketogenic diet and see what works best for you, but again, we lose weight when we are able to burn more calories than we are able to consume.

#2. Keto-Friendly Food & Sweeteners

When it comes to what you can and cannot eat on the ketogenic diet, people are still confused. There are either too few options or too many expensive alternatives, and then because fruits have too much sugar and vegetables have too many carbs some tend to believe these are the foods they should cut out during the ketogenic diet journey.

You should not cut out fruits and vegetables, especially the ones that are low in carbs and high in fiber—the latter especially is beneficial if you suffer from constipation.

Our other recommendation is that you remain focused on real food—so unprocessed as these usually contain all the extra and hidden carbs you want to avoid. Where possible, read the nutritional labels of the foods you buy and/or measure and calculate how much you can consume while still staying within the keto recommendations for carbs, protein, and fat.

Then there is the confusion and the debate about sweeteners.

One half says that sweeteners are the 'gateway' sticky sweet substance that could lead you back to carbs and unhealthy fats, thus throwing you off your keto lifestyle. The other half argues that they are more controlled than that, and if it weren't for the sweeteners, those keto-followers would not be able to comfortably commit to the diet.

Both are right because sweeteners can lead your body to have sugar cravings, but at the same time, sweeteners offer those on the diet the option of sweet, healthy treats to curb their cravings for non-keto-friendly food.

#3. Fat & Ketosis

Ketosis occurs in the body when the body has to burn fat instead of carbs for fuel, and this is a statement that leads some to believe that if they are not losing weight, it is because they are not consuming enough fats.

> One of the reasons keto diets work so well for weight loss is that they lower insulin levels and allow you to easily access your own fat stores for energy. This way of eating also helps you take in fewer calories by providing natural appetite suppression. (Spritzler, 2019, p. 136)

The solution here is to eat a little more protein, especially if you are consuming a less than moderate amount of this macro. The ketogenic diet does not consist of all the fats that we know and usually love but rather the healthy fats like olive oil, avocados, etc.

Do not make the mistake of consuming excessive amounts of fat without checking if they are heart-healthy and keto-friendly fats. Although, if you are still not losing weight after making these alterations, then try changing up your intake, the times that you eat, or try increasing your workout time or level of intensity.

#4. Yo-Yo Ketosis

Another misconception is that you can go back and forth on the ketogenic diet and be alright, which is a myth that is probably part of every diet and is so untrue.

Given the starting side-effects (keto flu, constipation, etc.) of the ketogenic diet, why would you even want to go back and forth? Once you are on the diet, stick to it, and if you are only temporarily on the diet, then stick to the diet until it comes time to end the diet. Also, when transitioning back to carbs, do so wisely and little-by-little to keep from overindulging and gaining back the pounds.

During the diet, you should wonder about the sort of healthy eating habits you would want to adopt into your life. Are you going to eat three times a day or five times a day? Are you going to eat all the carbs you missed during the diet or are you cutting some carbs out of your life for good? Are you still going to be drinking the correct amount of water or are you going straight back for fruit juices and all the other beverages that you might have missed during the ketogenic diet?

The ketogenic diet is an ideal time to ponder on these sorts of changes, a great way to practice healthy eating, and your chance to learn about limiting your calorie intake.

#5. Regarding Proteins

There are two misconceptions here; the first being that the ketogenic diet is all about protein, which it is not. The ketogenic diet is a low-carb, high-fat, and moderate protein diet. The second misconception is that too much protein can deter weight loss, but again, this is not true.

You should eat a moderate and the recommended (because our bodies are different) amount of protein. Too much protein can be turned to glucose and lead you to fall out of ketosis, while too little protein can lead to a larger appetite, decreased metabolic rate, and cause you to lose muscle mass.

Steps to the Ketogenic Diet

#1. Understand the Ketogenic Diet

As you've learned (and we delve a little deeper into this here), the keto diet recommends a daily macro intake of high fats, low carbs, and moderate protein (instead of the usual high carb, low fat, and moderate protein diet most people follow). With the restricted intake of carbs, the body is forced to burn fat instead of carbohydrates and ketones are generated in the body—in your liver, to be exact—and your body and brain use the ketones as their new source of energy.

However, this does not mean you can eat all the healthy fats in the world and still be burning fat, because your calories intake still matters.

On keto, weight loss is initially achieved from the water weight you lose due to the depletion of glycogen. Beyond that, your body burns both dietary and body fat, meaning that your excess fat stores are used, and this helps aid in weight loss. Further, due to the kinds of keto-friendly meals you will prepare, you will feel more satiated, leading you to feel fuller for longer, and thus, eat less or consume fewer calories.

The ketogenic diet encourages you to consume healthy fats and no starchy carbohydrates. Essentially, the ketogenic diet encourages you to practice a strict and healthy diet, which is why it works so well for so many individuals.

#2. Keto-Friendly Food

The next thing to do after knowing what to focus on is to learn about keto foods, which ones you can consume, which ones to avoid entirely, and which ones you can have occasionally.

On the ketogenic diet, the consumption suggestion we are given is that 55% to 60% of your daily meals should be fats and 5% to 10% should be carbs, and the remainder goes to protein. Although, again, everyone is different and needs certain amounts of macros, which is why we suggest you talk to a medically licensed dietician if you are ever unsure about how this restrictive diet will work for you.

However, simply put, you should only consume keto-friendly foods. Our next chapter will tell you more about the foods you can eat, cannot eat, and what you should be shopping for.

#3. Fatty Relationship

One of the things to do before committing to this diet is to consider your relationship with fat. As keto is the opposite of what you may be used to (high carb, low fat), you must look at your relationship with fat as you will be consuming much more of this. We have all heard that fat is bad for us, that fat clogs up our arteries to kill us, and as a result, a number of people are afraid of fat.

However, that is untrue, especially if you stick to healthy fats, which include avocados, certain nuts, nut butters, and olive oil (and some other options). If you happen to be the sort of person who is afraid of donuts and fries, that is okay, because those are not recommended on this diet and you can continue to stay away from those unhealthy foods.

If you are afraid of consuming even healthy fats (and in larger quantities), we recommend that you and fat become introduced quickly or at a pace you are comfortable with. How about reading up on some studies that illustrate the health benefits healthy fats have in store for you to get you started?

#4. Calculator

The three macronutrients are carbs, fats, and protein. Neither one of these macros should ever be completely cut out of your diet because then you may experience a nutrient deficiency, and this may lead to other illnesses. The low carbs you consume on keto offer you much-needed fiber, protein repairs the body, and fats suppress your appetite, plus, it is your main source of energy on keto.

When you start out on keto, you may need to learn to start tracking the number of macros you consume, and you do this by knowing how many calories you need. There are apps (MyFitnessPal, Cronometer, MyMacros+) that you can download on your phone or other smart device to track your calorie intake and your macros; however, you could also calculate your macros manually:

As you might remember, on the standard American diet, people consume 45% to 60% of their calories from carbohydrate sources, 20% to 35% from fats, and the remainder from protein. On the ketogenic diet though, the ratios are as follows

1. 5% to 10% from carbs
2. 60% to 75% from fat
3. 15% to 30% from protein

On a standard 2,000-calorie keto diet, here is how you can calculate how many grams of each macro you can consume per day. An important note: carbs and protein have 4 calories per gram, while fats have 9 calories per gram.

When we calculate the carbs: 2,000 x 0.05 = 100 carb calories. Divide this by 4 = 25 grams of carbs, which is your carb intake for the day, every day.

When we calculate the fats: 2,000 x 0.65 = 1,300 fat calories, divided by 9 = 144.44 grams of fat, which is your fat intake for the day, every day.

Lastly, we calculate the protein: 2,000 x 0.20 = 400 protein calories, divided by 4 = 100 grams of protein, which is your fat intake for the day, every day.

Until the diet becomes second nature, we recommend you only eat what you calculate and measure. Although this may seem like an inconvenience, it will certainly assist you in watching what you eat and will be better for you in general in the long run. This way, you can then also more easily make adjustments if you aren't losing weight or experience side effects.

#5. Clean House

Okay, so having only keto-friendly foods in your house is easier said than done.

You might be unsure which foods are keto-friendly and you may assume that all fruits and vegetables are the correct foods to be eating on a vegetarian keto diet but that is simply not true (more info on this coming soon so you know exactly what foods to keep, what to throw out, and what to add to your shopping list).

We suggest getting rid of any foods that may lead you astray, especially before you start the diet to help you exert control and stay on track. This is also helpful until you learn what to do when you have cravings or they disappear. Remember that we only experience cravings when our body wants a certain nutrient or mineral. Whatever your craving may be, there is a keto-friendly substitute that exists.

#6. Goals, Family, & Spotters

Another step to take towards the keto diet is considering your goals, sharing your plans with your family or friends, and getting someone to tag along or, at the very least, to 'spot' you.

Ask yourself now what do you want to accomplish with this diet and what do you see as the end result of your hard work, time, and sacrifices. You have to be realistic with your goals. Write down what you want to see, what habits you may want to implement in your life, and imagine the way you see yourself achieving your set goals. When we say things out loud, we often find the plot holes in our ideas and then we can make alterations where needed.

The reasons you chose to embark on this vegetarian keto journey are only known to you, but teamwork makes the dream work, so we suggest you talk to a family member or friends about your reasons. You could even ask a friend or a relative—one practiced in being committed and who would only motivate you to keep going—to tag along with you on the diet. Seriously, though, be wise and honest with yourself because you don't want to pick the friend who would sit with you on the couch and eat ice-cream with you on the days you feel like giving up; rather ask the friend who would remind you of your goals and the reasons giving up is not the answer.

If no one is willing to join you, you could ask them to be spotters, check on you every now and then, and you can go to them when you are having a hard time. Although, the best person to push you forward is you, so do the basic thing and get yourself a mantra and stick it above your mirror.

#7. **Determination**

Do not use your heart for this instead use your head.

Going into something just because it feels like the good thing or the right thing hardly guarantees results. You need to change your thinking and make the decision every day to persevere and remain determined, which is the right attitude to have.

Entering the diet with a goal in mind can only take you so far if you have the wrong attitude. You will need to adopt a 'will-do' attitude and remain committed and focused, even on the difficult days. You made an agreement with yourself to commit for a certain number of weeks or months and you cannot give up.

Are you ready to be totally and fully committed?

Okay, maybe committed is a big word because everything takes practice. There will be mistakes along the way, mistakes are excellent learning opportunities, and remembering everything you can and cannot do can be rather daunting at first. Although, with keto flu, we suggest you start this diet during a slow—not much going on—sort of week or over a long and chilled weekend.

During the first week, try to store only keto-friendly foods in the house, avoid that social gathering if you know you will be stuffing your face with processed foods by the end of the night, plan and calculate all your meals, and hydrate.

You could seriously use this diet as a chance to make some changes in your life. Note the bad habits that could be draining you or causing you to be unfocused about the other goals you want in your life. During this diet, you need to be tough on yourself and practice discipline.

We understand that some days are harder than others, and on those days, we recommend that you be honest with your spotter or someone who will understand. Talking things out can help you remember why keto-unfriendly food is a bad idea, it can also remind you of your goals, and talking out loud means you are louder than the voice in your head telling you to throw in the towel.

#8. Consider the Future

There are still some debates about the effects that the ketogenic diet can have as a long-term diet, but as we mentioned in our firsts chapters the same debate is still going on regarding the various vegetarian diets. The diet can be long-term or short-term depending on the person, but if you cannot live comfortably with a low amount of carbs, then make this a short-term keto diet.

Either way, you should still consider life after the diet or once you've settled into things. What sort of eating habits do you want to have once the diet is over? How often do you want to be eating on a daily basis?? What foods are you never going back to again? What foods are you excited to invite back into your life?

During the diet, note what is working for you and what is not working for you. Avoid going right back to a typical American diet and gaining back all the weight you lost. Truly consider what changes you would want to see in your life after the completion of this diet.

Burning Unwanted Fat

Sometimes, losing weight on the keto diet does not happen for some people, and we will now discuss if that could be because the diet isn't for them or if it is because they are doing something wrong. We are going to focus more on the things you could be doing wrong though if you aren't burning fat on the ketogenic diet and entering into a state of ketosis.

We will discuss the symptoms of the ketosis first.

There are the obvious symptoms, and the most obvious would be the *keto flu*, which we discussed in the previous chapter. The keto flu is a symptom of a changing diet but that is not the only symptom of ketosis.

Bad breath would be the first symptom, which is caused by a ketone—acetone—that exits in the body through the urine and the breath. The release of this ketone causes your breath to take on a more fruity smell.

Weight loss would be a clear and obvious sign that you are in ketosis, although during the first week, the weight you lose is considered to be stored carbs and water. However, seeing weight loss in the first week is a regular occurrence, and seeing yourself losing one to two pounds a week is another regular occurrence of the diet.

Decreased appetite is another symptom, which means you won't get as hungry as you used to or as often. Researchers say that this loss of appetite could be ketones 'telling' your brain to reduce your appetite.

Restlessness is the last symptom we are going to mention that has to do with ketosis; you may experience sleepless nights during the early stages of ketosis, but once your body gets used to things, you could even sleep better than before.

There are other symptoms like increased ketones in the blood and breath, increased focus and energy, fatigue and lowered performance, and digestive issues. Remember that if you are not seeing changes in your weight, these could be reasons:

#1. You could be eating too many carbs. You are supposed to limit your carbs to 5% to 10%. If you started the diet at 10% and you are not losing weight, then decrease your carb intake accordingly.

#2. You may not be eating foods that are not filled with enough nutrients or you may be snacking on

high-calorie foods. We suggest that you stick to whole foods and stay away from processed and fast food because they do not have the nutrients that you need, plus they may contain too many carbs. Also, in regard to snacks, although they may help with hunger between meals, try to limit the amount of snacks you consume in a week. Snacks and desserts are extra calories you do not need.

#3. You have not created a calorie deficit and that is one big way to lose weight on the ketogenic diet. Tracking, calculating, and measuring your calories help you create a deficit and so does working out. You cannot expect to lose weight if you are not watching what you eat and working out. Being physically active is important in any sort of diet. You can't expect to lose weight from just the way you eat; remember, you need to be burning more calories than the number of calories you consume.

#4. Another reason for not losing weight could be undiagnosed medical issues (depression, hypothyroidism, and high insulin levels). You could have a doctor check you out for any of these and you can move on with the diet from there. Another issue that could cause you to remain at the same weight is your stress levels and lack of sleep. Chronic stress causes the body to store up fat, which is the cause of that bulging belly.

#5. There is a quote on Pinterest (n.d.) about weight lost:

> It takes 4 weeks for you to notice a change. It takes 8 weeks for your friends to notice. It takes 12 weeks for the rest of the world to notice a change. It takes one day to decide that you are enough.

This was true for me; it may, however, not be true for you but this sure helped me to remain focused, and it reminded me that everything—no matter how much you want it or push at it—takes time. You may not have realistic weight loss goals, which could cause you to believe that nothing is happening; losing one to two pounds a week is healthy and within the range of what most people lose in that time frame.

The Bottom Line

After putting together the lists of myths surrounding the ketogenic diet, the things to consider before getting started on your vegetarian ketogenic diet, and what else to consider if you are not burning fat, we felt that journaling your progress would be of great assistance to you.

Journaling is one way to organize your thoughts—we are well aware that our thoughts can make or break us during our journey to healthy eating and weight loss. Our cravings begin as a thought that runs through our mind on a loop until we lose all reason why stuffing our faces with freshly made bread or warm chocolate chip cookies is a bad idea.

At the start of your journal, you could write down the reasons you are on the diet—seriously, it is hard to remember the reasons you need to stay on track on those really difficult days. Write what you expect from the diet and then rewrite your expectations if they are not realistic. During those difficult days, try journaling your thoughts and feelings over melting into the couch and stuffing your face with all the carbs you can find around the house.

And one of the beneficial things about journaling is being able to look back on the pages of your journal on other hard days and you will be reminded of why you are on this diet and remember all the days where you overcame and see how exactly you were able to subdue your cravings with keto-friendly foods.

We understand that journaling is not always for every person and, if that is the case, then you could try doodling, recording voice notes, video journaling, or simply listing your thoughts and feelings without providing any context, as long as you are aware of where you are on your journey and where you want to be at the end.

Always be honest and patient with yourself.

We trust this guide is able to encourage, enlighten, and assist you in getting started on a vegetarian keto diet. Remember to always keep your head held high—no false confidence here—and remain focused on the goals you want to accomplish.

Lastly, we believe your steps will be sure and your food will be measured!

Chapter 3: Vegetarian Keto Foods

This guide is specifically designed for lacto-ovo vegetarians on the *standard ketogenic diet,* and so we will follow the keto daily recommendations of 165 grams of fat, 40 grams of carbohydrates, and 75 grams of protein. For non-vegetarians who may be interested in combining the ketogenic diet and the vegetarian diet to lose weight or any other reason, this vegetarian keto diet is a meat-free diet (no animal flesh) and meat is not included in the list of foods to be consumed while on this diet or in the recipes.

We advise that you be aware of hidden carbs and read the nutrition labels (especially on processed and pre-packaged foods), especially at the start of the diet until you can be sure that whatever you are eating is keto friendly.

Our suggestion is that you avoid sugar, grains, starch, trans fats and hydrogenated fats, certain fruits, low-fat foods, and certain vegetables at all costs. There is a list of prohibited food below; however, there are some that need their own mentions.

Alcohol should be avoided, and if you can't, then alcohol intake should be limited to only hard liquor (rum, vodka, gin, etc.), low carb beer, and wine. Another suggestion is to avoid snacking and desserts, because these meals could slow down your weight loss; therefore, snack and enjoy dessert at your own discretion. If you do intend to consume snacks (and it is always good to be prepared with snacks in case the hunger bug bites) and dessert, we have some recipes for you to try. In regard to condiments, we suggest making your own when possible because most condiments are not keto-friendly (due to the extra carbs). Permitted condiments include reduced sugar ketchup, yellow mustard, keto-friendly ranch dressing, low-carb mayonnaise, vinaigrette dressing, and soy sauce.

Sweeteners like honey are not allowed at all but there are sweeteners like Stevia, sucralose, erythritol, monk fruit, yacon syrup, and xylitol that are keto-friendly and are safe to use. Always remember to check those nutrition labels and avoid artificial sweeteners.

We have arranged our lists into two categories— *forbidden and allowed foods* — in a list from A to Z.

The Forbidden Foods for a Vegetarian Keto Diet

The following is a list of foods you should try to avoid at all times during the vegetarian ketogenic diet. These foods are on this list because they are too high in carbs, and this can easily kick you out of ketosis. However, some of the food on this to-be-avoided list can, at times, be consumed in moderate amounts.

1. Agave. Apples. Apricots.
2. Bananas. Barbecue Sauce. Beans. Beer. Beetroots. Black Beans. Bread. Brown Sugar. Buckwheat.
3. Carrots. Cereal. Chickpeas. Cocktails. Cookies. Corn. Crackers.
4. Energy Drinks.
5. Granola. Grapefruit.
6. Honey. Honey Mustard.
7. Juice.
8. Ketchup.
9. Lentils.
10. Maple Syrup. Margarine. Marinades. Melon.
11. Oats. Oranges.

12. Parsnips. Pasta. Peanuts. Peas. Plums. Potato Chips. Potatoes. Pretzels.
13. Quinoa.
14. Rice. Rye.
15. Soda. Sports Drinks. Sweet Potatoes. Sweet Tea. Sweetened Salad Dressings.
16. Wheat. White Sugar. Wine.
17. Yams.

The Allowed Foods on the Vegetarian Keto Diet

Below is a list of foods you are allowed to consume on the ketogenic diet. Although, you should know that just because a food is permitted or has a low carb intake, does not mean you can eat as much of that food as you want.

- Aged Cheddar. Almond Butter. Almond Flour. Almonds.
- Baby Mushrooms. Blackberries. Blueberries. Brazil Nuts. Brie. Broccoli.
- Cabbage. Cauliflower. Chia Seed Meal. Coconut Flour. Cottage Cheese. Cream Cheese.
- Flaxseed Meal.
- Greek Yogurt. Green Beans. Green Bell Pepper.

- Half n' half. Hazelnuts. Heavy Cream.
- Macadamia Nuts. Mascarpone. Mayonnaise. Mozzarella.
- Parmesan. Pecans.
- Raspberries. Romaine Lettuce.
- Spinach.
- Tempeh. Tofu.
- Unsweetened Coconut.
- Yellow Onion.

The Weekly Grocery List

Listed below is everything you can purchase on the keto diet and these foods are vegetarian friendly. You can use this list as a basis of what to place in your shopping cart and what to leave behind. You can also determine your budget by going through this list to know what to buy. It would help if you planned your meals in advance to know what sort of food to always have in the house.

Beverages

- Almond milk

- Coconut milk
- Coffee
- Tea
- Water

Fruits

- Avocado
- Coconut
- Cranberries
- Lemon
- Lime
- Olives
- Raspberries
- Strawberries
- Tomatoes
- Watermelon

Vegetables

- Artichoke
- Arugula
- Asparagus
- Bell peppers
- Broccoli
- Cabbage

- Cauliflower
- Celery
- Collards
- Cucumbers
- Eggplant
- Garlic
- Lettuce
- Mushrooms
- Radishes
- Shallots
- Spinach
- Swiss chard
- Turnips
- Zucchini

The Fridge & Freezer Staples

- Apple cider vinegar
- Cauliflower rice
- Frozen berries
- Pickles
- Micro-greens
- Sauerkraut
- Sprouts
- Tempeh
- Tofu

Pantry Staples

- Almond flour
- Baking powder
- Baking soda
- Coconut flour
- Coconut milk (canned)
- Cocoa powder
- Dark chocolate (90%)
- Nutritional yeast
- Vanilla extract

Nuts & Seeds

- Almonds
- Brazil nuts
- Chia seeds
- Flax seeds
- Hazelnuts
- Hemp seeds
- Macadamia nuts
- Pecans
- Pumpkin seeds
- Sunflower seeds

Herbs & Spices

- Basil
- Cayenne Pepper
- Chili Powder
- Cilantro
- Cinnamon
- Cumin
- Oregano
- Parsley
- Rosemary
- Thyme

Nut & Seed Butters

- Almond butter
- Coconut butter
- Hazelnut butter
- Peanut butter
- Pecan butter
- Sunflower seed butter

Healthy Oils

1. Almond oil
2. Avocado oil
3. Coconut oil
4. Hazelnut oil
5. Macadamia nut oil
6. MCT oil
7. Olive oil

Sauces & Condiments

- Horseradish
- Hot Sauce
- Ketchup (no sugar added)
- Mustard
- Relish (no sugar added)
- Salad Dressings (no sugar added)
- Sauerkraut (no sugar added)
- Worcestershire Sauce

Sweeteners

- Erythritol

- Monk fruit
- Stevia
- Sucralose
- Xylitol
- Yacon Syrup

The Bottom Line

We are well aware that too often the issue with dieting is the purchasing of the above-mentioned products, which can be an expensive endeavor, and this is why we suggest you budget or even save up before starting. However, there are ways to start keto on a tight budget.

We understand that even thinking about how to get started or where to get the best deals could discourage you from giving this diet a real go. Top tips to get started on keto even when you don't have a large budget includes:

- Buying the groceries that will last longer in bulk
- Always looking for sales and shopping online to get better deals
- Buying fruits and vegetables that are in season

- Choosing the frozen fruits and vegetables over the fresh ones because they hold up better over long periods of time
- Planning your meals ahead of time so when you go to the store, you do not waste cash on food you think you need (and are not planned)
- Considering preparing your meals during the week in such a way that you will have leftovers that you can store for lunch the following day or dinner when you don't have time to cook.

Every person is different and, through the course of the diet, you will learn tips and tricks that work best for you. However, when it comes to cravings, we must think before we act; there are two things to consider:

Firstly, what is a keto-friendly substitute for what you are craving?

Secondly, is it the right time for you to be eating?

It sounds like a lot but take things at your own pace and try to learn one tip and trick at a time, as learning everything at once can be overwhelming. Through constant repetition and sticking to the vegetarian keto diet, you will learn to use these tips and tricks without even thinking about it.

Chapter 4: Keto-Friendly Fruits & Vegetables

Truthfully, for some of us—vegetarians—fruits and vegetables are our largest source of food, but because of the sugar in fruits and the carbs in vegetables, we are forced to remove some fruits and vegetables from our everyday diet if we want to follow keto.

Vegetables (especially those that grow underground) tend to have too much starch, fruits tend to have too much sugar, and together, they have too many calories that if consumed can cause you to fall out of ketosis. However, there are enough low-carb fruits and vegetables you can consume on the keto diet.

Keto-Friendly Fruits

Avocado

Nutrition Facts (100 grams)

Calories: 160

Fat: 15 grams

Carbohydrates: 9 grams

Protein: 2 grams

Originally, avocados come from south-central Mexico and are classified as a fruit even though the *botanically large berry* is used as a vegetable. The fruit is rich in vitamins, such as vitamin A, C, B-6, and magnesium.

Avocados are the most popular keto-friendly fruit out there, as they are included in so many of the recipes. They taste amazing, so it is totally understandable. Although, it is not only their taste that makes them so likable but also because they are rich in healthy fats.

Benefits of eating avocado include their ability to help combat heart disease and lower your cholesterol. Avos also improve insulin sensitivity, lower inflammation, and they contain more potassium than a banana (which is great, because you can't eat these yellow fruits while following keto).

At the end of the chapter, there is a wonderful *Keto Chocolate Ice Cream* recipe for you to try out, and the ice cream is made from avocados.

Blackberries

Nutrition Facts (100 grams)

Calories: 43

Fat: 0.5 grams

Carbohydrates: 10 grams

Protein: 1.4 grams

The blackberry comes from the Rosaceae family tree and is rich in vitamin A and C, calcium, iron, and magnesium. Blackberries are another keto-friendly fruit that you might not have thought about all that much, but you will be surprised to learn how much this little black fruit can do.

This fruit is rich in a number of vitamins that reduce inflammation, promote brain and motor function, healthy skin, and vitamins that slow the growth of cancer cells in the body.

Blackberries have also been used for years as a medicine, which is understandable given the fact that this fruit can do so much already on its own. Another amazing thing to note about blackberries is how rich they are in fiber, which means this fruit should be in great supply in your household at the start of your diet, because fiber can help with any gut issues you may have.

At the end of the chapter, there is a lovely blackberry inspired *Berry Pops* recipe that you can try out, which is another example of the tasty treats you can make with keto-friendly fruits.

Blueberries

Nutrition Facts (100 grams)

Calories: 57

Fat: 0.3 grams

Carbohydrates: 14 grams

Protein: 0.7 grams

Blueberries are native to North America, and are packed with vitamin C, vitamin A, iron, vitamin B-6, and magnesium. This is similar to the benefits of blackberries, which also promote healthy skin, brain and motor function, and your health in general.

Blueberries also assist in combating skin infections. However, blueberries contain the most carbs when compared to other keto-friendly berries, and so we suggest you limit your intake of this fruit.

Melons

Nutrition Facts (100 grams)

Calories: 30

Fat: 0,2 grams

Carbohydrates: 8 grams

Protein: 0,6 grams

Watermelons are farmed all over the world, but they originate from West Africa. The fruit contains vitamin A, vitamin C, and magnesium. The safest watermelons to have on the ketogenic diet is casaba melon, watermelon, cantaloupe, and honeydew melon, because they are low in carbs and have the least amount of sugar.

Honeydew melon fuels you throughout the day with its natural sugars, and it can boost your immune system, help keep your heart functioning the right way, and wash out toxins in the body that can cause illnesses.

Cantaloupe promotes healthy eye function, growth, and maintenance of cells in the body, as well as healthy teeth.

Watermelon, on the other hand, contains lycopene, which is an antioxidant that prevents cell damage and several types of cancer in the body. Other vitamins and minerals in the watermelon assist in boosting cardiovascular health.

Nevertheless, melon is another fruit you have to be careful with on the ketogenic diet; ensure you measure and calculate your intake of carbs.

Raspberries

Nutrition Facts (100 grams)

Calories: 53

Fat: 0,7 grams

Carbohydrates: 12 grams

Protein: 1,2 gram

Raspberries come from the Rubus plant, which is a plant of the rose family, and they are filled with vitamin C, calcium, iron, magnesium, and vitamin B-6. This tiny red fruit is also packed with antioxidants that fight against inflammation. Raspberries contain a high polyphenol content and this can help reduce blood pressure and prevent plaque building up in the arteries.

Starfruit

Nutrition Facts (100 grams)

Calories: 31

Fat: 0,3 grams

Carbohydrates: 7 grams

Protein: 1 gram

Averrhoa carambola is a tree that can be found in tropical sectors around the world and grows star fruit. Star fruit or carambola consists of vitamin C, magnesium, and vitamin A.

This fruit is keto-friendly. It looks like a lemon and bell pepper combo, and has a sweet and sour taste to it. The star fruit is anti-inflammatory and heart-friendly, regulates blood pressure, and promotes weight loss.

Strawberries

Nutrition Facts (100 grams)

Calories: 33

Fat: 0,3 grams

Carbohydrates: 8 grams

Protein: 0,7 grams

Strawberries is our second last fruit on this list. The fruit is grown and enjoyed on a world-wide scale, and it is classified as a hybrid species of the genus Fragaria. The strawberry is rich in vitamin C, iron, magnesium, and calcium.

Strawberries are beneficial when it comes to blood sugar levels, insulin levels, and in promoting insulin sensitivity. Although, be wise about how many strawberries you consume and how often you consume them because you don't want to risk falling out of ketosis.

Tomatoes

Nutrition Facts (100 grams)

Calories: 18

Fat: 0,2 grams

Carbohydrates: 3,9 grams

Protein: 0,9 grams

Originally, tomatoes came from western South America and Central America. Tomatoes are rich with vitamin C, potassium, folate, and vitamin K.

The tomato is a fruit used too often as a vegetable and not just in the ketogenic diet. There is also the antioxidant lycopene in tomatoes, the same antioxidant found in watermelons, and it promotes heart disease and cancer.

At the end of the chapter, there is a tasty *Tomato Soup* recipe you can try out and enjoy on those chilly winter nights.

Keto-Friendly Vegetables

When it comes to vegetables, the best and safest are the above ground vegetables. Underground vegetables generally contain too many carbs, especially potatoes and sweet potatoes, so say goodbye to those crispy fries and mashed potatoes.

Onions are another major no-no, but because we mainly stick to the spice (onion powder) and we do not generally consume all that many onions, they are permitted. However, it would be better to use scallions or green onions if you really need to use an onion in a recipe. Know and research your alternatives, especially if you are developing a non-ketogenic recipe into a vegetarian keto-friendly one.

Another recommendation is to stick to the red bell peppers as the green and yellow have a higher carb count. If you are ever unsure about which vegetables to pick, then always go for green and leafy ones.

We can summarize that above ground, green, and leafy vegetables are our safest bet. One exception is corn.

Asparagus

Nutrition Facts (100 grams)

Calories: 20

Fat: 0,1 grams

Carbohydrates: 3,9 grams

Protein: 2,2 grams

The young shoots of asparagus are used as spring vegetables. The vegetable contains vitamin A, vitamin C, iron, and vitamin B-6. Asparagus promotes blood clotting, bone health, cell growth, and DNA formation.

You can try baking and melting cheese over your asparagus, or you could roast or cook this vegetable and pair it with a keto-friendly sauce or other dinner meals.

Bell Pepper

Nutrition Facts (100 grams)

Calories: 31

Fat: 0.3 grams

Carbohydrates: 6 grams

Protein: 1 gram

Bell peppers come in a variety of colors, from green, orange, white, yellow, red, and purple. Bell peppers are packed with vitamin A, vitamin C, magnesium, and vitamin B-6, and the green bell peppers contain the lowest number of carbs.

You could stuff your peppers with a compatible ingredient of your choice or chop them up into your breakfast eggs or add color to your fried cauliflower rice recipe.

Broccoli

Nutrition Facts (100 grams)

Calories: 34

Fat: 0,4 grams

Carbohydrates: 7 grams

Protein: 2,8 grams

Broccoli is part of the cabbage family and filled with vitamin C, vitamin A, vitamin B-6, and magnesium. Broccoli is a fun green vegetable that can be steamed or roasted and/or covered in cheese. The vegetable is crunchy and filled with so much flavor.

There are several ways to enjoy broccoli but there is a *Roasted Broccoli* recipe for you to try out at the end of the chapter.

Cauliflower

Nutrition Facts (100 grams):

Calories: 25

Fat: 0,3 grams

Carbohydrates: 5 grams

Protein: 1,9 grams

Cauliflower is an annually grown plant, which is packed with vitamin C, vitamin B-6, and magnesium. The cauliflower is a vegetable you should always have in the house, because there are so many things you can make with cauliflower. You can use it as a rice and mash it or even chopped it into chicken-like bits. You can really play around with this vegetable.

There is a great *Hash Browns* recipe at the end of this chapter in which you can use your cauliflower.

Green Beans

Nutrition Facts (100 grams)

Calories: 31

Fat: 0,1 grams

Carbohydrates: 7 grams

Protein: 1,8 grams

Green beans are part of the bean family and are a source of vitamin C, vitamin B-6, magnesium, iron, and calcium. These veggies are good for your eyes, heart, and digestion.

Green beans are quite enjoyable and can be enjoyed as an excellent side-dish with any of your dinner meals; and they can be enjoyed steamed or roasted.

Lettuce

Nutrition Facts (100 grams)

Calories: 15

Fat: 0,2 grams

Carbohydrates: 2,9 grams

Protein: 1,4 grams

Lettuce is part of the daisy family and offers you vitamins like vitamin A, vitamin C, iron, calcium, vitamin B-6, and magnesium. This leafy hydrating vegetable is low in calories, promotes weight loss, and is packed with antioxidants.

There are different kinds of lettuce (iceberg, butter, radicchio, romaine, kale, and many others) you can use in your meals for crunch and for a heightened flavor, and yes, lettuces can be used for more than just salads.

Mushrooms

Nutrition Facts (100 grams)

Calories: 22

Fat: 0,3 grams

Carbohydrates: 3,3 grams

Protein: 3,1 grams

Mushrooms are classified as a fungus that is packed with vitamin C, iron, vitamin B-6, and magnesium. This veggie is an immune system booster and the antioxidants in the vegetable combat things like heart disease and cancer.

Mushrooms can be chopped and thrown in the frying pan, glazed with garlic sauce and paired with some bell peppers and eggs, or added to cauliflower rice for extra taste.

Spinach

Nutrition Facts (100 grams)

Calories: 23

Fat: 0,4 grams

Carbohydrates: 3,6 grams

Protein: 2,9 grams

Originally, this leafy green vegetable came from central and western Asia. Spinach is packed with calcium, magnesium, and vitamin A. This vegetable is low in carbs and high in nutrients, which makes it one of the best vegetables to always have around.

The best way to enjoy spinach is as a creamy side-dish, so check out the recipe at the end of this chapter, and add your own little twist to it if you want.

Zucchini

Nutrition Facts (100 grams)

Calories: 17

Fat: 0,3 grams

Carbohydrates: 3,1 grams

Protein: 1,2 grams

A zucchini is classified as a summertime squash. The cucumber-looking vegetable is filled with vitamin C, iron, vitamin B-6, and magnesium. Zucchini aid in weight loss and promote healthy digestion.

There are a number of recipes you can find that use zucchini on the vegetarian keto diet like fries and chips. You can grill, fry, and grate zucchini for use in your recipes.

Keto-Friendly Veggie & Fruit Recipes

Keto Chocolate Ice Cream

Keto Chocolate Ice Cream is the bittersweet ice cream that offers you the chance to indulge in a sweet but healthy treat.

Ensure that the ingredients you use are keto-friendly and that they are low in sugar.

The recipe below yields 6 servings. Although, you can alter it to one serving in case you are easily tempted to overindulge.

Note: if you do not have an ice cream maker, then no worries; our instructions below cover another way to still make this recipe.

Time: 12 hours

Serving Size: 1 bowl

Prep Time: 4 hours

Cook Time: 8 hours

Nutritional Facts/Info:

Calories: 216.17 grams

Carbs: 3.72 grams

Fat: 19.38 grams

Protein: 3.86 grams

Ingredients:

- 25 drops liquid Stevia
- 6 squares unsweetened chocolate
- 2 large avocados
- 2 tsp. vanilla extract
- 1 cup coconut milk
- ½ cup heavy whipping cream
- ½ cup unsweetened cocoa powder
- ½ cup powdered erythritol

Directions:

1. You are going to need to blend the avocado, coconut milk, cream, and vanilla extract in a blender until fully combined. The mixture should be smooth and lime green in color.
2. Add the powdered erythritol, liquid Stevia, and cocoa powder to the creamy mixture, and blend together until fully combined.

3. Break the unsweetened chocolate squares into chunky pieces and add to the coffee brown creamy mixture, and freeze together in a medium-large bowl for 8 hours.
4. Use the freeze and stir method to get that creamy ice cream texture and you are going to need to put the ice cream in a shallow dish container for this part.
5. Put the ice cream in the freezer for 30 minutes, then remove and stir the ice cream, and then put the ice cream back in the freezer for 30 minutes.
6. You should repeat the above-mentioned action for 3 hours, until the ice cream starts sticking and molding to the container.
7. Once the process is complete, you can serve and enjoy.

Berry Pops

Berry Pops are popsicles you can make with the use of blueberries and raspberries —two major keto-friendly fruits. This is an ideal dessert recipe that even your non-keto following family and friends will enjoy.

A few notes for this recipe:

- You will need popsicle molds and sticks.

- You can substitute the coconut cream with the whole cream.
- If you want to use strawberries instead of raspberries or blueberries, check the intake of macros first.

When you start freezing the molds, use the times as suggestions because some freezers—like mine—do not freeze liquids quickly enough, so allow for extra time if you have the same issue with your freezer.

The recipe below yields 6 Berry Pops.

Time: 5 hours

Serving Size: 1

Prep Time: 3 hours

Cook Time: 2 hours

Nutritional Facts/Info:

Calories: 146.33

Carbs: 5.26 grams

Fat: 13.07 grams

Protein: 1.14 grams

Ingredients:

- 1 ½ tsp. liquid Stevia

- 1 ½ cup canned coconut cream
- 1 cup frozen raspberries
- 1 cup frozen blueberries
- 1 cup water
- ½ tsp. vanilla extract

Directions:

1. You will need to use two small- to medium-sized pots to set to boil at medium-high temperature. In one pot, you will cook the raspberries, ½ cup of water, and ½ tsp. of liquid Stevia together. In the second pot, you will need to cook ½ cup of water, ½ tsp. of liquid Stevia, and blueberries.
2. Both of the raspberries and the blueberries mixtures should boil for 5 minutes before you can take them off the stove. Allow the mixtures to cool slightly—you do not want the heat to crack your glass blender if you transfer the too-hot liquid in the blender.
3. Blend the raspberry and blueberry separately until smooth and pour them out into separate bowls before allowing them to cool in the fridge.
4. Use a jug (this makes it easier for pouring) or a small bowl to mix together the coconut cream, ½ liquid Stevia, and vanilla extract. Put the mixture in the fridge for later use.
5. Imagine a traffic light for the next part, well if the green light was red (raspberry mixture), the

yellow light was white (coconut cream mixture), and the red light was blue (blueberry mixture). You would need to layer and fill your molds in the same way.

6. Scoop 3 tbsp. of raspberry mix into the molds and put the mold in the freezer for 1 hour.
7. Scoop 4 tbsp. of coconut mix into the same mold once the raspberry has set and put the mold in the freezer for 30 minutes.
8. Insert sticks into each mold; the coconut mix should be semi-set to properly hold the sticks, and put the mold back in the freezer for 1 hour.
9. The last 3 scoops to be placed into the mold is the blueberry mixture; after you have scooped the blueberry mix into the mold, place the mold back into the freezer for a maximum of 2 hours.
10. And once the pops have set, you can enjoy your tasty summer-time fruity dessert.

Tomato Soup

Tomato Soup is exactly what you need on those cold winter nights when you just want to hug a bowl of warm soup to your chest.

The recipe below can make 4 bowls of Tomato Soup.

Time: 35 minutes

Serving Size: 1 bowl

Prep Time: 10 minutes

Cook Time: 25 minutes

Nutritional Facts/Info:

Calories: 301.5

Carbs: 8.75 grams

Fat: 25.79 grams

Protein: 9.29 grams

Ingredients:

1. 1 x 6 oz. can of tomato paste
2. 1 cup heavy whipping cream
3. 1 tsp. oregano
4. 1 tsp. garlic powder
5. ½ tsp. kosher salt
6. ¼ cup water
7. ¾ cup shredded parmesan cheese

Directions:

1. First, you will need a medium-sized pot. Place this on the stove and set the plate to a low-medium heat.
2. Shortly after that, throw in the tomato paste and garlic and stir the ingredients together until they are smoothly combined.

3. Once the tomato paste and garlic are combined, add the cream to the mix, which will lighten the color of the soup, and stir until the soup begins to simmer.
4. When the soup starts to bubble, you can add in the cheese, a teaspoon full at a time until the soup starts to thicken, at which point you can pour in ¼ cup of water and cook the soup for another 5 minutes.
5. You can serve immediately or reheat for later enjoyment.

Roasted Broccoli

Roasted Broccoli is an excellent side dish that could be paired with some fried cauliflower rice or another keto-friendly dinner meal. They are also so quick and easy to make, so you do not even have to wonder if they will be worth your time to pair with your meal.

This recipe makes a total of 6 servings, and the leftovers can be stored in a sealable container in the freezer and reheated for other meals, although they won't be as crunchy.

Time: 30 minutes

Serving Size: 1

Prep Time: 5 minutes

Cook Time: 25 minutes

Nutritional Facts/Info:

Calories: 138.17

Carbs: 5.24 grams

Fat: 10.77 grams

Protein: 4.83 grams

Ingredients:

- 3 tsp. garlic powder
- 2 tbsp. chopped fresh basil
- 1 ½ pound broccoli florets
- ⅓ cup Parmesan cheese
- ½ tsp. kosher salt
- ½ tsp. red chili flakes
- ½ lemon juice and zest
- ¼ cup olive oil

Directions:

1. Turn on the oven and set the temperature to 425 degrees Fahrenheit.
2. Use silicone baking pads to cover the bottom of your baking tray, lay the broccoli florets out on the tray, and drizzle the broccoli with olive oil, freshly chopped basil, garlic powder, kosher

salt, red chili flakes, lemon zest (grated lemon skin), and lemon juice.

3. Shower the broccoli with Parmesan cheese and put the tray in the oven for 25 minutes before serving right out of the oven for your enjoyment.

Low-Carb Cauliflower Hash Browns

Low-Carb Cauliflower Hash Browns are a great breakfast dish on their own, but they can also be a wonderful breakfast side-dish. You could pair them with anything or, as is traditional, top them off with some sour cream or fried scallions.

These hash browns are crunchy, keto-friendly, and easy to throw together and make.

You should use a keto-friendly butter if you want to use butter, which you can drizzle over the hash browns when done, but in this recipe, we make use of olive oil for frying.

This recipe yields 4 servings you can store in the fridge in a sealable container.

Time: 25 minutes

Serving Size: 1

Prep Time: 10 minutes

Cook Time: 10 minutes

Nutritional Facts/Info:

Calories: 331

Carbs: 8.5 grams

Fat: 31.9 grams

Protein: 7.3 grams

Ingredients:

- 16 oz. of cauliflower
- 1 small onion
- 3 large eggs
- 1 tsp garlic salt
- Pinch of pepper
- 8 tbsp of olive oil

Directions:

1. Start by washing your vegetables and then proceed by breaking the cauliflower into florets and blending them in your food processor. They should resemble little grains of white fluffy rice.
2. Next, grate your onion and add it to the cauliflower before adding the mix to a medium-sized bowl. Add in the eggs, garlic salt, pepper,

and any other seasoning of your choice, and mix together before setting the mixture aside for 10 minutes.
3. During the 10 minutes that the mixture sets, you can start pouring olive oil into a medium heated frying pan.
4. Scoop out the hash brown size you want into the frying pan; do not turn the hash brown too early, rather wait until it is golden brown on one side or else it may crumble.
5. Each side of the hash brown should be fried for 3 to 4 minutes and you can add more oil to the frying pan if needed.
6. Finally, once the hash browns are cooked, you can enjoy them with your own choice of toppings.

Creamy Spinach

Creamy Spinach consists of spinach and a creamy Parmesan and cream cheese mixture, which is the essence of this delicious side meal.

The recipe below yields 3 servings and the leftovers can be stored in the fridge and reheated in the microwave for another meal.

Time: 20 minutes

Serving Size: 1

Prep Time: 5 minutes

Cook Time: 15 minutes

Nutritional Facts/Info:

Calories: 165

Carbs: 3.63 grams

Fat: 13.22 grams

Protein: 7.33 grams

Ingredients:

1. ¼ tsp. onion powder
2. 10 oz. frozen spinach
3. 3 oz. cream cheese
4. 3 tbsp. Parmesan cheese
5. 2 tbsp sour cream
6. ¼ tsp. garlic powder

Directions:

1. Take the spinach out of the freezer and allow the spinach to defrost at room temperature through the day.
2. Cook the spinach in a saucepan on a medium heat until the excess water from the spinach has dried out.

3. Sprinkle the spinach with garlic powder, onion powder, and any other seasoning of your choice.
4. Now, stir in the cream cheese and allow the cream cheese to melt into the spinach before adding the sour cream into the spinach, and then melting the Parmesan into the spinach.
5. Stir the creamed spinach for another 2 minutes before serving as a side dish.

The Bottom Line

You have got options!

We hope you have learned for the last two chapters. You have tons of food options and ideas to try out; however, you must be willing and ready to get into the kitchen and learn to prepare your own meals.

The best way to partake in a vegetarian ketogenic diet is learning to prepare your own foods, which should also encourage you to come up with new tasty recipes that could expand the options we have as vegetarians.

However, there are wonderful recipes that are part of this chapter that you can try out. You could alter them to meet your needs; they are really tasty and worthwhile.

But don't think there are just six recipes for you! The next couple of chapters are jammed-packed with tasty recipes for you to try out.

Chapter 5: Vegetarian Keto Diet Breakfast Ideas

Blueberry Pancakes

Blueberry Pancakes are low in carbohydrates and quite an excellent and an enjoyable breakfast. The golden pancakes are light and fluffy and not too sweet. You can pair the pancakes with a keto-friendly syrup, but these pancakes are pretty tasty on their own.

What you are going to need to make these pancakes is a large mixing bowl, an electric mixer, a ladle, a spatula, measuring cups and spoons, and lastly, your trusted pancake-making pan, which is just my way of referring to a non-stick pan. When it comes to short-term storing of the pancakes, you can place the pancakes in a sealable container and store them in your fridge, but for long-term storage, it is better to keep them in your freezer and defrost them in the microwave.

The recipe yields 4 Blueberry Pancakes.

Time: 12 minutes

Serving Size: 1

Prep Time: 10 minutes

Cook Time: 2 to 3 minutes on each side or until golden brown.

Nutritional Facts/Info:

Calories: 389.25

Carbs: 7.23 grams

Fat: 33.26 grams

Protein: 19.05 grams

Ingredients:

- 3 large eggs
- 1 cup almond flour
- 1 tsp. baking powder
- ½ tsp. vanilla extract
- ½ cup golden flaxseed meal
- ¼ cup unsweetened vanilla almond milk
- ¾ cup ricotta cream
- ¼ tsp. salt
- ½ tsp. Stevia powder
- ¼ cup blueberries

Directions:

1. Set the above-mentioned ingredients out on the kitchen counter, take out your measuring cups and spoon, and start by whisking the three eggs until frothy in your mixing bowl.
2. Pour vanilla extract, ricotta cream, and the almond milk to the eggs and gently mix the ingredients together with an electric whisk.
3. Proceed by adding Stevia, almond flour, and baking powder into the bowl, gently whisk the ingredients together, then add in the flaxseed meal and salt, and whisk until smooth.
4. Set the mixture aside.
5. Now, place the pan on the stove and set the temperature to a medium heat, and while you wait, cut your berries in half.
6. Check the heat of the pan by sprinkling some water in it, and if the water sizzles, then you can add a small amount of butter to grease the pan.
7. Use a ladle to pour the pancake mixture into the hot pan, place 6 halved berries on the pancake, and use a spatula to flip the pancakes when the edges begin to brown.
8. Repeat the above process to make three other pancakes.
9. Once done, place the yellow-golden pancakes on a plate, and top them off with a keto-friendly topping of your choice.

Low-Carb Brownie Muffins

Low-Carb Brownie Muffins are a yummy breakfast to make and have on-the-go, and with a yield of 4 tasty and chewy muffins, you can already save the other two for the next day's breakfast, thus saving time and money.

What you are going to need to make this high fiber breakfast muffin is a large mixing bowl, an electric mixer, measuring cups and spoons, and your keto-friendly ingredients.

You can store any remaining muffins in a sealable container and enjoy these later.

Time: 25 minutes

Serving Size: 1 muffin

Prep Time: 10 minutes

Cook Time: 15 minutes

Nutritional Facts/Info:

Calories: 289.5

Carbs: 6.55 grams

Fat: 21.14 grams

Protein: 10.47 grams

Ingredients:

- 2 tbsp. coconut oil
- 1 cup golden flaxseed meal
- 1 tbsp. cinnamon
- 1 large egg
- 1 tsp. vanilla extract
- 1 tsp. apple cider vinegar
- ¼ cup cocoa powder
- ½ tbsp. baking powder
- ½ tsp. salt
- ¼ cup sugar-free caramel syrup
- ½ cup pumpkin purée
- ¼ cup slivered almonds

Directions:

1. Start by turning the oven on and setting the temperature to 350 degrees Fahrenheit.
2. Break the egg into the large mixing bowl, add in the coconut oil and caramel syrup, and blend using the electric mixer. The mixture will be yellow in color and have a sticky texture.
3. Now pour in the vanilla extract, apple cider vinegar, and pumpkin purée and whisk together with the mixer. The mixture should still be yellow but more watery in texture.
4. Mix in the cocoa powder, flaxseed, cinnamon, slivered almonds, and salt to the yellow

mixture, and combine until the mixture is brown and grain-like in texture.
5. Spray your muffin pan with non-stick baking spray or grease four muffin molds with coconut oil. Scoop the mixture into the 4 molds and bake the muffins for 12 to 15 minutes.
6. Allow the muffins to cool before removing them from the molds and enjoying right away.

Veggie Scramble

Veggie Scramble is the crunchy and fluffy egged morning breakfast. Our recipe is bursting with colors and flavors and really fantastic spices.

You can use other keto-friendly vegetables and spices for this scramble. For example, you can substitute the eggs with more thinly sliced baby mushrooms.

This recipe makes 2 dishes.

Time: 25 minutes

Serving Size: 1

Prep Time: 15 minutes

Cook Time: 10 minutes

Nutritional Facts/Info:

Calories: 311

Carbs: 4.9 grams

Fat: 24.5 grams

Protein: 14.2 grams

Ingredients:

- ¼ cup olive oil
- ¼ red onions
- ½ tsp. salt
- ½ tsp. turmeric powder
- 1 cup chopped spinach
- 1 tbsp. coconut milk
- 1 tsp. cayenne pepper
- 1 tsp. garlic powder
- 4 baby mushrooms
- 4 eggs
- 4 mini bell peppers

Directions:

1. Start by placing a pan on the stove at a low-medium heat and pour olive oil in the pan.
2. Cut the baby mushrooms into slices, chop the spinach, red onions, and bell peppers, and place the ingredients in the pan to fry until onions or peppers start to brown around the edges.

3. Use a small-medium bowl to beat the eggs until foam starts to form, whisk in the coconut milk and salt, and add the mixture to the pan and scramble the ingredients together until the eggs are cooked to your liking.
4. Add the turmeric, cayenne pepper, and garlic powder to the mix, cook for 5 minutes and scramble with a fork, and dish it out right away and serve.

Keto Breakfast Granola

Keto Breakfast Granola is the crunchy morning breakfast you will enjoy with that full-fat and no-sugar Greek yogurt. There will also be enough left over from this recipe to have for your breakfast for at least a week and a half to two weeks.

Talking about leftovers, you can store the granola in the fridge to ensure it remains crispy and crunchy. You can also swap in the nuts for your own choice of nuts but ensure you don't overindulge.

The recipe below yields 15 Keto Breakfast Granola servings.

Time: 25 minutes

Serving Size: ½ cup

Prep Time: 5 minutes

Cook Time: 35 minutes

Nutritional Facts/Info:

Calories: 169

Carbs: 5 grams

Fat: 16 grams

Protein: 4 grams

Ingredients:

- 5 tablespoon coconut oil
- 3 cups coconut flakes
- 1 cup raw macadamia nuts
- ½ cup raw almonds
- ¼ walnuts
- ¼ pumpkin seeds
- 2 tsp. chia seed
- 1 tsp. cinnamon powder

Directions:

1. Turn the oven on to 250 degrees Fahrenheit.
2. You can chop your almonds, macadamia, and walnuts, or you can blend them together in your food processor.

3. Pour the nuts into a bowl and mix in the pumpkin and chia seeds, cinnamon powder, coconut flakes, and coconut oil together until nicely combined.
4. Proceed with lining a baking tray with wax paper and then spread the nuts and seeds out on the tray.
5. Place the tray in the oven for 35 minutes and rotate the nuts halfway through.
6. Remove the tray from the oven and cool before serving with keto-friendly yogurt or toppings of your choice.

Mixed Berry Smoothie

This keto mixed berry smoothie is a truly *sweet* way to start your morning.

A mixed berry smoothie does not seem like the greatest idea in the world when you are on the keto diet; however, the secret is to choose the correct berries. Strawberries and raspberries are keto-friendly, but you can throw in some blackberries for extra flavor.

Nevertheless, to thicken the smoothie, you could throw in ice cubes or avocados. And you can add some chia seeds in there too for extra thickness and more nutrient benefits.

Time: 5 minutes

Serving Size: cup

Prep Time: 5 minutes

Nutritional Facts/Info:

Calories: 388

Carbs: 13.1 grams

Fat: 38.3 grams

Protein: 3.9 grams

Ingredients:

- 3 cubes of ice
- ¼ cup of mixed berries (raspberry, strawberry, and blackberry)
- ½ tsp erythritol (optional)
- ⅔ cup of coconut milk

Directions:

1. Blend ice cubes for 10 seconds in the blender or until crushed.
2. Now add in the raspberries, strawberries, blackberries, erythritol, and coconut milk into

the blender and combine until smooth and pink.
3. Serve chilled, and you can sprinkle some chia seeds on top.

Low-Carb Oatmeal

Low-Carb Oatmeal can cure that oatmeal craving that you may have.

This is a quick and easy to make breakfast meal that is high in protein, moderate in fat, and low in carbs, so it is a great after-workout breakfast meal and totally worth your time.

You could either use a keto-friendly milk of your choice or stick to water for this recipe. The recipe below serves one person, but if you wish to make extra, then simply double the ingredients by the amount of people you want to serve.

Furthermore, this meal is higher in carbs, so ensure you stay within your macro counts with regard to your meals the rest of the day.

Time: 8 minutes

Serving Size: 1 bowl

Prep Time: 1 minute

Cook Time: 5 minutes

Nutritional Facts/Info:

Calories: 274

Carbs: 21.7 grams

Fat: 18.4 grams

Protein: 9.5 grams

Ingredients:

- ½ cup of coconut milk
- 3 tbsp of almond meal
- 1 tbsp of coconut flour
- 1 tsp of chia seeds
- ½ of cinnamon

Directions:

1. Pour the coconut milk into a small pot, set the temperature on the stove to a medium heat, and allow the milk to simmer.
2. Stir in the almond meal, coconut flour, chia seeds, Stevia, and cinnamon.
3. Allow the oatmeal to boil for 1 minute at the same heat before dishing out into a breakfast bowl.

Chapter 6: Vegetarian Keto Diet Lunch Ideas

Collard Green Veggie Wraps

Collard Green Veggie Wraps are a mouthwatering lunch and also a dinner option. They are bursting in veggie colors, crunchy and scrumptious, and the tzatziki sauce makes you wish every meal tasted this good.

Imagine sushi but the fish is collard green leaves, and the stuffing is cucumber, red bell pepper, purple onion, Kalamata olives, feta cheese, and cherry tomatoes.

There is so much flavor in this one lunch meal for you to enjoy! You can prepare the wraps the night before and store it in a sealable container before placing the container in the fridge for later use.

With the recipe below, you can make 4 servings of Collard Green Veggie Wraps.

Time: 25 minutes

Serving Size: 1 wrap

Prep Time: 25 minutes

Cook Time: N/A

Nutritional Facts/Info:

Calories: 165.34 grams

Carbs: 7.36 grams

Fat: 11.25 grams

Protein: 6.98 grams

Ingredients:

1. 2.5 oz. cucumber
2. 2 tbsp. olive oil
3. 2 tbsp. minced fresh dill
4. 1 cup full-fat plain Greek yogurt
5. 1 tsp. garlic powder
6. 1 tbsp. white vinegar
7. 8 Kalamata olives
8. 4 large collard green leaves
9. 4 cherry tomatoes
10. 1 medium cucumber
11. ½ medium red bell pepper
12. ½ cup purple onion
13. ½ block feta

Directions:

1. You will begin by making the tzatziki sauce, which you should store in the fridge for later use, and you are going to need a small- to medium-sized bowl for this.
2. Grate the cucumber on a cutting board first to ensure the excess water from the cucumber is not mixed into the tzatziki.
3. Transfer the cucumber into the bowl, then add in the olive oil, minced fresh dill, full-fat plain Greek yogurt, garlic powder, and white vinegar. Stir the ingredients together until they resemble a white paste.
4. And now for the wrap, you will need to wash all the ingredients for the wrap.
5. Cut the Kalamata olives and cherry tomatoes in half.
6. Dice the purple onion and cut the feta cheese into one-inch thick strips.
7. Cut the cucumber and red bell pepper into strips (like fries).
8. Cut the stems off the collard green leaves and thickly 'butter' each leaf with tzatziki sauce.
9. Proceed with topping the leaves with the cucumber slices, then the pepper, onion, olives, feta, and the tomatoes in the center of the wrap. Fold the wraps like a burrito (fold the sides and then fold the middle).

10. Cut the wraps in half and use the rest of the sauce on top of your wraps for extra deliciousness.

Red Pepper Spinach Salad

Red Pepper Spinach Salad is a great light lunch salad to have on those days where you need to keep your calorie count down, so you can maybe enjoy some keto chocolate ice cream for dessert without the guilt.

This is a quick and easy meal to make and to enjoy on those really busy days.

The recipe below yields 2 servings of Red Pepper Spinach Salad.

Time: 10 minutes

Serving Size: 1 bowl

Prep Time: 10 minutes

Cook Time: N/A

Nutritional Facts/Info:

Calories: 212.68

Carbs: 5.01 grams

Fat: 19.49 grams

Protein: 6.5 grams

Ingredients:

- 6 cups spinach
- 3 tbsp. Parmesan cheese
- 1 tsp. red pepper flakes
- ¼ cup ranch dressing

Directions:

- Throw together the spinach and the ranch dressing in a bowl until nicely combined.
- Once the spinach and ranch are combined, then mix in the Parmesan cheese and sprinkle the mix with red pepper flakes.
- Serve and enjoy.

Keto Club Salad

Keto Club Salad is so worth to diet for!

Imagine a bowl filled to the rim with red, yellow, green, and white. This is a truly filling lunch meal with a satisfying crunch.

The recipe below should provide you with 3 servings, and you can store any leftovers by sealing them in a container and putting the container in your fridge.

Time: 35 minutes

Serving Size: 1 bowl

Prep Time: 15 minutes

Cook Time: 20 minutes

Nutritional Facts/Info:

Calories: 329.67

Carbs: 4.83 grams

Fat: 26.32 grams

Protein: 16.82 grams

Ingredients:

- 4 oz. cheddar cheese
- 3 large eggs
- 3 cups iceberg lettuce
- 2 tbsp. sour cream
- 2 tbsp. mayonnaise
- 1 tsp. dried parsley
- 1 ½ tbsp. milk
- 1 cup cucumber
- 1 tbsp. Dijon mustard
- ½ tsp. garlic powder

- ½ tsp onion powder
- ½ cup cherry tomatoes

Directions:

1. Start by getting out all the above-mentioned ingredients, a medium-sized bowl, a cutting board, and a small-medium pot.
2. You should lay everything you need on a clean kitchen counter top and ensure you thoroughly wash your vegetables.
3. Firstly, pour some water into the pot, put the pot on medium heat on the stove, put the eggs in the water, cover the pot, and allow the eggs to harden in the water. The suggested time is about 9 minutes for a medium-sized egg, 12 minutes for a large egg, and longer for bigger eggs.
4. While the eggs are boiling, start cutting your vegetables on the cutting board. Start by tearing the iceberg lettuce to pieces, cut the cheddar cheese into cubes, cut your cherry tomatoes in half, and dice your cucumber.
5. Place every ingredient in the bowl once you are done cutting, tearing, and dicing them.
6. The eggs should be boiled at this point, so remove the pot from the plate, and pour cold water from the tap into the pot so the eggs cool down much quicker and they stop cooking.
7. While you wait on the eggs to cool, make the dressing by stirring together, in a small bowl,

the sour cream, mayonnaise, milk, garlic powder, onion powder, and dried parsley. The dressing should not be too watery. Store in the fridge for later use.
8. And now you can peel the eggs, cut them in half, and place them in the bowl with the rest of the salad.
9. Stir your salad, mixing the colors together, squirt some Dijon mustard in the center of the salad, and coat the salad in the dressing.
10. Cover the leftovers and store in the refrigerator.

Grilled Cheese Zucchini

Grilled Cheese Zucchini is not exactly as weird as it sounds; the zucchini is the sandwich and man, does the zucchini taste like the best darn keto-friendly sandwich ever. You are seriously going to enjoy this crispy and crunchy filling 'sandwich.'

What you are going to need is a spatula, frying pan, cutting board, and all the ingredients listed below.

This recipe makes 3 servings, so you can make one 'sandwich' to enjoy now and store the rest away for another day in the week, therefore, saving you time and money.

Time: 25 minutes

Serving Size: 1 'sandwich'

Prep Time: 10 minutes

Cook Time: 15 minutes

Nutritional Facts/Info:

Calories: 300

Carbs: 4 grams

Fat: 14 grams

Protein: 20 grams

Ingredients:

- 2 cup grated zucchini
- 2 cup shredded cheddar
- 2 green onions
- 1 large egg
- ½ cup freshly grated Parmesan
- ¼ cup cornstarch
- ½ tsp. basil powder
- A pinch of salt and pepper
- Olive oil

Directions:

1. Wash your zucchini before grating 2 cups worth of zucchini onto your cutting board, then grate the Parmesan cheese into a mixing bowl, and add the zucchini to the same mixing bowl.
2. Whisk your egg in a small bowl with salt, pepper, and basil; then add this mix into the mixing bowl of zucchini and Parmesan.
3. Cut your onion into thin slices and add the onion slices and cornstarch to the mixing bowl before mixing the ingredients together. The mixture should resemble a white batter.
4. Now, take your frying pan, put it on the stove, set the temperature on the plate to a medium heat, and pour enough olive oil to cover the pan.
5. Use a spoon and flatten out 4 tablespoons of the batter onto the pan, and form these into a square.
6. Fry the zucchini on both sides until golden, and then move the zucchini to a plate, fry another slice, and repeat the action until you have the amount of Grilled Cheese Zucchini 'slices' that you want.
7. Place a cooked zucchini back on the pan, spread cheddar or your cheese of choice onto the zucchini, and place another cooked zucchini on top. Wait for the cheese to melt before flipping over, and do this for all your other zucchini 'slices' and fry each for a 1 or 2 minutes.

8. Place the 'sandwich' on a plate, cut in two, and enjoy.

Asparagus Fries

Asparagus Fries is a great snack, an equally amazing side dish, and easy lunch time meal. The majority of fat (42.57 grams) in this recipe comes from the 3 tbsp of mayonnaise. The 10 medium asparagus spears contain 6.21 grams of carbs and 3.4 grams of fiber, and the ½ cup of shredded Parmesan cheese provides the most protein at 15.14 grams.

Ensure your mayonnaise is keto-friendly, but if you don't, you can make homemade mayonnaise with the provided ingredients below.

The recipe makes a total of 2 servings, and the homemade mayonnaise amounts to 1 ¼ cups worth of mayonnaise.

Time: 30 minutes

Serving Size: 1

Prep Time: 20 minutes

Cook Time: 10 minutes

Nutritional Facts/Info:

Calories: 453.65

Carbs: 5.51 grams

Fat: 33.43 grams

Protein: 19.14 grams

Ingredients: Asparagus Fries

- 10 medium asparagus spears
- 3 tbsp. mayonnaise
- 2 large eggs
- 2 tbsp. chopped parsley
- 1 tbsp. roasted and chopped red pepper
- ½ cup shredded Parmesan cheese
- ½ tsp. garlic powder
- ½ tsp. smoked paprika
- ¼ cup almond flour

Ingredients: Mayonnaise

- 3 drops liquid Stevia
- 2 large egg yolks
- 1 large egg
- 1 tsp. Dijon mustard
- ½ cup melted coconut oil
- ¾ cup olive oil
- A pinch of salt
- A pinch of smoked paprika

Directions:
- Preheat the oven to 425 degrees Fahrenheit.
- Unless you have a keto-friendly mayonnaise, start by making your mayonnaise: soften the coconut oil in the microwave, which should take 20 to 60 seconds. Shortly after that, pour and mix the olive oil in a small-medium bowl.
- Pour egg yolks, liquid Stevia, egg, Dijon mustard, salt, and smoked paprika into your blender, blend the ingredients, and add the oil in little by little (drops) until the mayonnaise *emulsifies*, and only after that can you start adding the oil more frequently between pulses.
- Transfer the mayo to a sealable container and you can keep it in the fridge. The mayo will last for a maximum of 3 weeks. If you want the mayo to last for much longer, you will need to add 1 tbsp. of whey to the mix and allow they mayo to set for roughly 8 hours before you can refrigerate it.
- You are going to need to use a small-medium container to combine the chopped roasted red pepper and mayonnaise together. Allow the mayo pepper mix to chill in the refrigerator.
- And now take the Parmesan cheese, parsley, and garlic powder and place these ingredients in your blender, and mix until smooth. Add the ¼ cup of almond flour, and mix until the mixture resembles bread crumbs.

- Pour the mixture onto a kitchen tray and season the mixture with the smoked paprika.
- Whisk the eggs in a medium-sized container (you will need to be able to coat the asparagus in this bowl, so ensure the container is large enough for this process) until the eggs start to foam.
- Now coat the asparagus in the egg mix, then you have to hold the asparagus over the 'bread crumb' mixture and sprinkle the mixture over the asparagus.
- Transfer every piece of asparagus straight to the baking tray after coating them in the 'bread crumb' mixture, and once all the asparagus has been coated, pour any leftover mixture over the asparagus in the tray.
- Place the tray in the oven and bake for 10 minutes or until the 'bread crumbs' begin to brown.
- After taking the asparagus out of the oven, you can begin consuming your crispy warm fries with your homemade red pepper aioli.

Avocado Taco

Avocado Taco is an amazing and flavorful lunch or even a dinner time dish, filled with healthy good fats, and a hearty combo of nuts and vegetables.

And what you are going to need for this is a grinder, a frying pan, as well as the yummy keto-friendly ingredients listed below.

There should be enough taco filling for two avocados, so you can save the leftover taco filling in a sealable bag and store in your freezer for lunch during the week or to have the same dinner later in the evening.

Time: 20 minutes

Serving Size: ½ avocado

Prep Time: 10 minutes

Cook Time: 10 minutes

Nutritional Facts/Info:

Calories: 454

Carbs: 6.5 grams

Fat: 40 grams

Protein: 16 grams

Ingredients:

1. 1 cup raw walnuts

2. 1 tbsp. hulled hemp seeds
3. 1 tsp. cumin
4. 1 tsp. garlic powder
5. 1 tsp. salt
6. ½ cup chopped onion
7. ½ medium avocado
8. 3 tbsp. shredded cheddar cheese
9. 2 tsp. adobo sauce
10. 4 tsp. smoked paprika
11. 4 tbsp. avocado oil
12. 7 oz. cauliflower

Directions:

1. Get out all the above-mentioned ingredients and start by cutting your onion into thin slices and placing them in the grinder with cauliflower florets, raw walnuts, hemp seeds, cumin, garlic powder, and lastly, the salt or a seasoning of your choice.
2. Place a large pan on the stove and set it to a low temperature, and add in 2 tbsp. of avocado oil.
3. Grind the ingredients together until the mixture you see in your grinder resembles tiny bread crumbs. Note: if your pan isn't large enough to fit in the mixture, then divide the mixture in two.
4. Set the temperature on the pan to a medium heat and add in the mixture, use a spatula or wooden spoon for stirring, and cook 2 to 4

minutes before adding 2 tbsp. adobo sauce (if you are only cooking half, then use 1 tbsp. of adobo sauce).
5. Cook for 5 more minutes; the taco filling should be brown in color and look like minced meat. Add in the 2 tbsp. of cheddar cheese (1 tbsp. if cooking in halves).
6. Cut your avocado in 2 and remove the seed.
7. Dig out enough space in your avocado for the taco filling, stuff the avocado with the taco filling you just made, and top the filling with 1 tbsp. of cheddar and the previously dug out avocado.

Mushroom & Avocado Salad

Mushroom & Avocado Salad is another amazing lunch time meal, and the buttered mushrooms really ties the entire meal together.

You are seriously going to enjoy this flexible meal that allows for all sorts of alterations and add-ins. What you are going to need to make this dish is a pan, spatula, and the ingredients you can find in the list below.

The recipe below makes one bowl of Mushroom & Avocado Salad.

Time: 15 minutes

Serving Size: 1

Prep Time: 5 minutes

Cook Time: 10 minutes

Nutritional Facts/Info:

Calories: 617

Carbs: 7 grams

Fat: 55.7 grams

Protein: 17.5 grams

Ingredients:

- 1 avocado
- 1 oz. goat cheese
- 1 tbsp. balsamic vinegar
- 1 tbsp. butter
- 1 tbsp. olive oil
- 2 oz. cremini mushrooms
- 4 oz. spring mix
- Salt and pepper

Directions:

1. Start by gathering all the ingredients and crumbling your goat cheese, cutting the avocado into small cubed pieces, and cutting the mushrooms into slices.
2. Now, place your pan on the stove and set the temperature to a medium heat.
3. While you wait for the pan to warm up, take a bowl and pour in the spring mix, crumbled cheese, and cubed avocados.
4. Place 1 tbsp. of butter in the pan and add the mushroom in. Once the butter has melted, and sprinkle with salt and pepper. Allow the mushrooms to cook until golden brown and add them to the salad.
5. Use a small bowl to combine 1 tbsp. of olive oil and 1 tbsp. of balsamic vinegar.
6. Coat the salad with the olive oil balsamic vinegar combo, mix the salad together, and you can dig into a delicious lunch time salad.

Chapter 7: Vegetarian Keto Diet Dinner Ideas

Keto Broccoli Salad

Keto Broccoli Salad is a great dinner option that allows you to get all your healthy and keto-friendly veggies in for the day.

There are so many fun flavors and colors in this one dish that it is darn near inspiring. Essentially, this is the meal that could make you really content with eating healthy.

You can opt to cook the broccoli in boiling water for five minutes on a medium heat or eat the broccoli raw. You could also use thinly chopped almonds instead of pumpkin seeds.

The recipe yields 8 servings.

Time: 25 minutes

Serving Size: 1

Prep Time: 25 minutes

Cook Time: N/A

Nutritional Facts/Info:

Calories: 357.13

Carbs: 3.95 grams

Fat: 32.01 grams

Protein: 12.11 grams

Ingredients:

- ½ cup pumpkin seeds
- ½ medium red onion
- ¾ cup mayonnaise
- 1 large avocado
- 3 cups broccoli florets
- 3 tbsp. apple cider vinegar
- 4 oz. cheddar cheese
- 5 tablespoon erythritol
- Salt and pepper

Directions:

- In a small container, mix together the mayonnaise, erythritol, and the apple cider vinegar to make the dressing for the salad.
- Set the dressing aside and wash your vegetables, and on a cutting board, cut the

broccoli into bite-size pieces and place the pieces in a medium-large sized bowl.
- Dice half of a red onion and add it to the bowl.
- Cut your cheddar into cubes and add to the bowl.
- Then cut your avocado into slices, then cut the slices in three, and add them to the mix.
- Pour the dressing over the bowl and combine the vegetables.
- Serve and enjoy.

Zucchini Skins

Zucchini Skins can be used for a quick and easy to make keto dinner, or it can even be made and served as an appetizer.

You may substitute the squash for another low carb keto-friendly squash.

Three zucchini is worth 11.01 grams of carbs and 3.5 grams of fiber, the 2 oz. of cheddar is worth 18.89 grams of fat, and 2 oz. of pepper jack cheese contains 13.88 grams of protein.

When it comes to storing the zucchini skins, you can place them in a sealable container in the fridge and use the microwave to reheat them prior to serving.

The recipe yields 6 servings worth of zucchini skins.

Time: 35 minutes

Serving Size: 6

Prep Time: 15 minutes

Cook Time: 20 minutes

Nutritional Facts/Info:

Calories: 108.5

Carbs: 2.82 grams

Fat: 8.25 grams

Protein: 5.76 grams

Ingredients:

- 3 small Zucchini
- 3 whole diced baby mushrooms
- 3 tbsp. sour cream
- 2 tsp. smoked paprika
- 2 oz. shredded cheddar cheese
- 2 oz. shredded Pepper Jack cheese
- 2 tbsp. chopped chives
- 1 tsp. olive oil
- 1 tbsp. Worcestershire sauce
- 1 ½ tsp salt

Directions:

1. Start by cutting the squashes right down the middle into six even halves; imagine them as little boats, and carve the seeds out of the zucchini with a spoon before sprinkling the slices with 1 tsp. of salt.
2. Next, you need to turn on your oven and set the temperature to 375 degrees Fahrenheit.
3. Use a small-medium container to prepare the diced mushrooms by dressing the mushrooms with the oil, smoked paprika, Worcestershire sauce, and ½ tsp. of salt.
4. On a baking tray, lay out the zucchini and mushrooms, place the tray in the oven, and allow it to cook until lightly browned.
5. Once you have taken the tray out of the oven, you can layer the zucchini with mushrooms, jack cheese, and the cheddar cheese.
6. Place the tray back in the oven and take the tray out of the oven once the cheeses begin to melt, and enjoy the meal with some sour cream sprinkled with chopped chives.

Tofu & Bok Choy

Crispy Tofu & Bok Choy Salad is a tasty and crispy lunch time meal with a wonderful salad dressing. The majority of the fat (40.42 grams) in this recipe comes from the 3 tbsp. of coconut oil; 9 ounces of bok choy is worth 5.56 grams of carbs and 2.5 grams of fiber. The 3 tbsp. of soy sauce contain 3.91 grams of protein.

Some tips or alternatives for this recipe:

- You can substitute the monk fruit extract with Stevia.
- Remember to use a keto-friendly peanut butter.
- Also, you will need to dry out your tofu, which will take about 6 hours. Try drying the tofu the day before, then marinate the tofu through the night. In the morning, you can place the tofu in the oven to bake and put the recipes together for your lunch. Store the leftovers in a sealable container and store away in your fridge. However, you can only store the crispy tofu for 3 days. When it comes to reheating the crispy tofu, you can use the microwave, but the tofu will not retain its crispiness. Therefore, we suggest using the oven and reheat the tofu at a temperature of 375 degrees Fahrenheit.
- The bok choy salad can be refrigerated for roughly five days. Store the leftover tofu, bok choy, and sauce separately, which will make it easier to reheat the tofu in the oven.

This recipe makes 3 servings.

Time: 8 hours 35 minutes

Serving Size: 1 bowl

Prep Time: 8 hours

Cook Time: 35 minutes

Nutritional Facts/Info:

Calories: 398.59

Carbs: 6.68 grams

Fat: 30.43 grams

Protein: 24.11 grams

Ingredients: Oven Baked Tofu

- 15 oz. extra firm tofu
- 2 teaspoons minced garlic
- ½ a lemon
- 1 tbsp. soy sauce
- 1 tbsp. sesame oil
- 1 tbsp. water
- 2 tsp. garlic powder
- 1 tbsp. rice wine vinegar

Ingredients: Bok Choy Salad

1. 9 oz. ok choy
2. 7 drops liquid monk fruit extract
3. 3 tbsp. coconut oil
4. 2 tbsp. chopped cilantro
5. 2 tbsp. soy sauce

6. 1 tbsp. sambal oelek
7. 1 stalk green onion
8. 1 tbsp. peanut butter
9. ½ a lime

Directions:

1. Dry out your tofu with the assistance of two clean kitchen towels. First, lay the kitchen towel on a plate or kitchen tray, lay the tofu on the towel, put the second towel on top of the tofu, and then lay some heavy books —that you will not need for the next 6-hour processes—on top of the towel.
2. Once the tofu has been dried out with the use of towels, you need to fry-dry the tofu: cut the tofu into even slices, lay the slices out on a non-stick pan (no oil), and fry until the tofu is light brown in color. Cut the tofu into evenly sized squares.
3. Use a medium-sized container for the flavoring: mix together the soy sauce, sesame oil, water, garlic, vinegar, and lemon juice.
4. In a sealable plastic bag, toss the tofu squares and the flavoring you just made together, and allow the flavors to soak in for 2 hours.
5. Once the tofu has marinated in the flavoring for the allotted time, proceed by preheating the oven at a temperature of 350 degrees Fahrenheit.

6. Line your baking tray with wax paper, lay the tofu on the tray, and bake in the oven for a maximum of 35 minutes or until the tofu is golden brown in color.
7. While the tofu is in the oven, cut the bok choy into small slices.
8. Continue by stirring together the chopped green onion and cilantro, coconut oil, soy sauce, sambal oelek, peanut butter, lime juice, and monk fruit extract in a small-medium bowl to make the salad dressing.
9. Once you remove the tofu from the oven, you can make your Crispy Tofu & Bok Choy Salad by combining the tofu, bok choy, and sauce together.
10. Now get your chopsticks and enjoy.

Grilled Eggplant

Grilled Eggplant is a dinner dish with an amazing tasty sauce that really brings some true flavor to the grilled eggplant.

You are going to need a grill for this meal. Although the grilled eggplant is best served when warm, you can still store it in foil and refrigerate for serving the next day.

Our recipe only serves two but you can double the amount of eggplant to make extra and share with your non-vegetarian friends or family members. We are sure they will especially enjoy the tahini dressing.

Time: 30 minutes

Serving Size: 1

Prep Time: 20 minutes

Cook Time: 10 minutes

Nutritional Facts/Info:

Calories: 298

Carbs: 36.1 grams

Fat: 15.6 grams

Protein: 11.8 grams

Ingredients:

- 1 large eggplant
- 3 tbsp lemon juice
- 2 tbsp parsley
- ½ olive oil
- 1 tsp dried oregano
- ¼ tsp red pepper flakes
- A pinch of sea salt
- A pinch of black pepper
- ⅓ cup of tahini

- 2 tbsp water
- 1 tbsp garlic

Directions:

1. Use a medium-sized bowl to mix together tahini, lemon juice, water, and garlic, to make the tahini dressing, and then cover the bowl before putting it aside.
2. Use a medium-high heat for the grill. While the grill heats up, you can mix together the oil, oregano, and red pepper flakes in a small bowl.
3. Slice the eggplant into ¼--inch slices and lather the slices with the oil-oregano-pepper-flakes mix, and then place the slices on the grill.
4. Cook the slices for 3 minutes on each side or until golden yellow.
5. Lastly, drizzle the tahini dressing over the eggplant and enjoy.

Caprese Salad

Caprese Salad is a real summer time salad and a tasty Italian dish.

The is filled with the juices from grape tomatoes, the softness of mozzarella, and the healthy fats of avocado. What you are going to need for this meal is a serving bowl, a spoon, and the ingredients of course.

Time: 20 minutes

Serving Size: 1

Prep Time: 10 minutes

Cook Time: 10 minutes

Nutritional Facts/Info:

Calories: 284

Carbs: 8 grams

Fat: 26 grams

Protein: 6 grams

Ingredients:

- 1 cup balsamic vinegar
- ¼ cup extra virgin olive oil
- ¼ tsp. garlic powder
- ¼ tsp. sea salt
- ⅛ tsp. black pepper
- 2 cup grape tomatoes
- 1 cup mozzarella balls
- 1 medium avocado
- ⅓ cup fresh basil

Directions:

- Start with cutting the grape tomatoes in half, dice the avocado, and chop the basil.
- Put the tomatoes, avocado, and basil in a medium-sized bowl, and in another bowl, mix together the balsamic vinegar, olive oil, garlic powder, sea salt, and black pepper.
- Add the balsamic olive oil mix to the bowl of tomatoes, avocado, basil and mix these together to ensure the salad is properly dressed.
- Serve in a bowl and save any leftovers for later.

Broccoli Creamy Casserole

Broccoli Creamy Casserole is an enjoyable dinner time dish with keto-friendly vegetables, like cauliflower and broccoli, to create lovely colors and tasty flavors. As you go through the recipe, you may notice that the minced 'meat' is the same as the taco filing in the lunch chapter for the Avocado Taco recipe. Well, it is a great tasty mix that works as our minced 'meat' for his broccoli creamy casserole.

You can cook your broccoli first before putting it in the oven, but cook your broccoli in such a way that the crunchiness won't be lost unless it is something that doesn't matter to you.

The recipe below yields 8 servings.

Time: 1 hour 10 minutes

Serving Size: ⅛ Casserole

Prep Time: 10 minutes

Cook Time: 60 minutes

Nutritional Facts/Info:

Calories: 441

Carbs: 16.18 grams

Fat: 31.3 grams

Protein: 20.2 grams

Ingredients: Minced 'Meat'

- 1 cup raw walnuts
- 1 tbsp. hulled hemp seeds
- 1 tbsp. cheddar cheese
- 1 tsp. adobo sauce
- 1 tsp. garlic powder
- 1 tsp. onion powder
- 1 tsp. salt
- 2 tbsp. avocado oil
- 2 tsp. smoked paprika
- 4 oz. cauliflower

Ingredients: Broccoli Creamy Casserole

- ¼ tsp. rosemary
- ¼ tsp. thyme
- ½ cup mayonnaise
- ½ tsp. dried basil
- ½ tsp. smoked paprika
- 1 cup plain full-fat Greek yogurt
- 1 cup shredded cheese
- 1 tsp. garlic salt
- 1 tsp. onion powder
- 14 oz. bags frozen broccoli
- 8 oz. cream cheese

Directions:

1. Preheat the oven to 350 degrees Fahrenheit and wash your broccoli and cauliflower.
2. Start by placing your cauliflower florets in the blender with raw walnuts, hemp seeds, cumin, garlic powder, onion powder, and salt or a seasoning of your choice.
3. Grind the ingredients together until the mixture you see in your grinder resembles tiny bread crumbs.
4. Place a pan large on the stove and set it to a low temperature and add in 2 tbsp. of avocado oil.
5. While you wait for the pan to heat, place broccoli florets, cream cheese, Greek yogurt, mayonnaise, garlic salt, onion powder, dried basil, smoked paprika, rosemary, and thyme in a large mixing bowl.

6. Now, return to the minced 'meat' and set the temperature on the pan to a medium heat and add in the mixture. Use a spatula or wooden spoon for stirring, and cook 2 to 4 minutes before adding 2 tbsp. adobo sauce.
7. Cook for 5 more minutes; the minced 'meat' should be brown in color and look like browned minced meat. Add in the 2 tbsp. of cheddar cheese.
8. Dish the minced 'meat' into the same mixing bowl as the broccoli, and use a wooden spoon to combine the ingredients.
9. Then grease your casserole dish before dishing the contents of the mixing bowl inside, and drizzle the shredded cheese on top before transferring the casserole to the already heated oven.
10. Cook the casserole for a maximum of 50 minutes or until the cheese begins to bubble.
11. Remove the dish from the oven, cut into eight equal pieces, dish out the needed amount, serve, and cover and store the rest in the refrigerator.

Cauliflower Broccoli Stir Fry

Cauliflower Broccoli Stir Fry is an amazing dinner meal that is pretty easy to make, and it is another cauliflower and broccoli combo with red bell peppers and mushrooms, which are our keto-friendly vegetables. That just shows you how much you can do when you limit your diet to only nine vegetables.

What you are going to need for this recipe is a frying pan, wooden spoon, and measuring cups and spoons.

The recipe below yields 4 servings for you to absolutely enjoy. You can cover the leftovers and store them in the fridge for later use.

Time: 20 minutes

Serving Size: 1

Prep Time: 10 minutes

Cook Time: 10 minutes

Nutritional Facts/Info:

Calories: 126

Carbs: 8.8 grams

Fat: 7.6 grams

Protein: 4.2 grams

Ingredients:

1. ¼ cup soy sauce
2. ½ medium red bell pepper
3. ½ tsp. red pepper flakes
4. 1 medium onion
5. 1 tbsp. avocado oil
6. 1 tbsp. ginger
7. 2 tsp. sesame oil
8. 2 whole garlic cloves
9. 3 oz. cremini mushrooms
10. 4 ounces cauliflower
11. 7 oz. broccoli

Directions:

1. Start with washing all your vegetables, then on a cutting board, peel and grate the ginger, mince the garlic, chop the onion, cut the red bell pepper into slices, cut the mushrooms into slices, and break the cauliflower and broccoli into florets (tiny broccoli and cauliflower trees).
2. Place the different ingredients in separate bowls and put every other ingredient aside except for the garlic, ginger, soy sauce, vinegar, and cauliflower florets.
3. Coat the cauliflower florets thoroughly in the garlic, ginger, soy sauce, and vinegar. Allow the flavors to really sink in by setting the bowl of marinating florets aside.
4. Pour 1 ½ tbsp. of avocado oil into a wok or frying pan that is set on a low-medium heat

and throw in onion. The onion should be a light faint brown before you can add in the red bell pepper, mushrooms, and broccoli.
5. Stir the ingredients in the pan together and, once the broccoli and the red bell pepper start to brown, add in the cauliflower and another 1 ½ tbsp. of avocado oil. Note: do not throw away the marinade.
6. Cook the ingredients together for roughly 5 minutes or until the cauliflower browns and pour in the marinade into the wok to be stirred with the ingredients in the pan until the sauces have almost evaporated.
7. Dish the food out into a bowl and dig right in.

Chapter 8: Vegetarian Keto Diet Snack Ideas

Keto Cucumber Sushi

Keto Cucumber Sushi is a cucumber stuffed with other vegetables, so there is no need to worry because there is no fishy business going on here. The snack is crunchy and refreshing and can be used as a side dish.

Time: 20 minutes

Serving Size: 1

Prep Time: 15 minutes

Cook Time: N/A

Nutritional Facts/Info:

Calories: 190

Carbs: 9 grams

Fat: 16 grams

Protein: 1 gram

Ingredients:

- 2 carrots
- 1 cucumber
- 1 tbsp. sriracha
- 1 tsp. soy sauce
- ½ red bell pepper
- ½ yellow bell pepper
- ⅓ cup mayonnaise
- ¼ avocado

Directions:

1. In a small bowl, whisk the mayonnaise, sriracha, and soy sauce to make the dipping sauce, then put the sauce in the fridge.
2. The next thing to do is cut your avocado, carrots, and bell peppers into slices.
3. Cut your cucumber in two and use a teaspoon to hollow out the center. Use a butter knife to spread avocado around the inside of the cucumber.
4. Stuff the cucumber with bell peppers and carrots until the cucumber is packed with the vegetables.
5. Lastly, slice the cucumber into one-inch thick pieces and enjoy with the sauce.

Avocado 'Potato' Chip

Avocado 'Potato' Chip is another one of those weird sounding recipes, but it is really not. This is a salty, healthy, and enjoyable snack that even your friends might be interested in. You can store the leftovers in a jar in the pantry or a sealable bag in the pantry.

The recipe yields 16 chips.

Time: 45 minutes

Serving Size: 1

Prep Time: 10 minutes

Cook Time: 35 minutes

Nutritional Facts/Info:

Calories: 120

Carbs: 4 grams

Fat: 10 grams

Protein: 7 grams

Ingredients:

1. ½ tsp. garlic
2. ½ tsp. Italian seasoning

3. ¾ cup freshly grated Parmesan
4. 1 large ripe avocado
5. 1 tsp. lemon juice
6. Salt and pepper

Directions:

1. Start by preheating your oven to 325 degrees Fahrenheit.
2. Cut the avocado in two, dish it into a medium bowl, and mash the avocado with a fork until it is smooth in texture.
3. Add the Parmesan, lemon juice, garlic powder, basil, oregano, rosemary, and salt. Lay parchment paper on the baking sheet.
4. Use a teaspoon to place the mixture on the baking sheet and space out. Use the teaspoon to flat the scoop.
5. Bake for 30 minutes and wait for the chips to cool before digging in.

Strawberry Milkshake

Strawberry Milkshake is another one of the great treats you can make with keto-friendly fruit like strawberries. You can enjoy this recipe as a snack or dessert. Every sip is cooling and sweet but keto-friendly nonetheless.

The majority of the fats (21.47 grams), carbs (1.63 grams), and protein (1.69 grams) comes from the ¼ cup of heavy whipping cream.

The recipe yields only 1 serving; try not to overindulge.

Time: 5 minutes

Serving Size: 1 glass

Prep Time: 3 minutes

Cook Time: 2 minutes

Nutritional Facts/Info:

Calories: 368

Carbs: 2.42 grams

Fat: 38.85 grams

Protein: 1.69 grams

Ingredients:

1. 7 ice cubes
2. 2 tbsp. sugar-free strawberry Torani (or sugar-free strawberry syrup)
3. 1 tbsp. MCT oil
4. ¾ cup coconut milk (from the carton)

5. ¼ tsp. xanthan gum
6. ¼ cup heavy cream

Directions:

1. Start blending the 7 ice cubes in the blender.
2. When the ice is crushed pour in your syrup, MCT oil, milk, xanthan gum, and heavy cream and blend the ingredients together until smooth and soft pink in color.
3. Serve in a tall glass and prepare to have your taste buds lose their tiny minds!

Mixed Berries Fruit Roll Ups

Mixed Berries Fruit Roll Ups are the ideal snack time idea. Growing up with fruit roll ups and dried fruit, this recipe was exciting for me to make, and you are seriously going to love these.

You can try the recipe with other keto-friendly fruits or the ones that are low enough in carbs to try out; you know, the fruits you should only enjoy occasionally.

Nevertheless, what you are going to need for this recipe is a strainer, a spoon, a bowl, a silicone mat, and a baking pan. You are going to use an oven to dry out your fruit roll up, but if you have a dehydrator, you can use that too.

The recipe below produces 8 pieces of fruity fruit roll ups.

Time: 5 hours 15 minutes

Serving Size: 1

Prep Time: 15 minutes

Cook Time: 5 hours

Nutritional Facts/Info:

Calories: 14

Carbs: 7.5 grams

Fat: 0.2 grams

Protein: 0.3 grams

Ingredients:

- 1 tbsp. lemon juice
- 3 tbsp. erythritol
- 1 cup raspberries
- 1 cup strawberries

Directions:

1. Start with washing your raspberries and strawberries, then cut the stem of your

strawberries and cut each strawberry into four pieces.
2. You are going to purée your berries into a bowl with a strainer and large spoon, although if you've got a blender or food processor, then you can use those, but our process purées and removes the seeds from the berries at the same time.
3. Place the chopped strawberries in the strainer, let the strainer hover over a small- to medium-sized bowl, and press the strawberries until all the juices have been drained out.
4. Now, rinse out the strawberry seeds from your strainer and now purée the raspberries in the same way you did with the strawberries. You can cut the raspberries if you think it will make things easier.
5. Once both berries have been puréed into the same bowl, add in the erythritol and 1 tbsp. of lemon juice. Stir the ingredients together until fully combined.
6. Proceed by turning on your oven and setting the temperature to 140 degrees Fahrenheit.
7. Place a silicone mat on your baking pan, gently pour the pure on the mat, and use a clean spoon to even it out, and then cook it in the oven for 3 to 5 hours. When it is ready, the center of the dried purée should not be sticky.
8. You should carefully peel the fruit roll up from the silicone and cut it into the shape and

number of pieces you want, or cut eight strips out and roll them up and secure them with tape.
9. Note that the fruit roll up will be dry but will get sticky overnight, so be sure not to place them too close together in case they stick to one another.
10. You can enjoy the roll ups after they have completely set (i.e., gotten sticky).

Low Carb Pumpkin Spice Fat Bombs

This recipe is ideal for individuals on-the-go and those who would not be able to live without the taste of pumpkin spice. You will be able to meet your fat intake needs with these little treats.

You are sure to have fun making these and can either use a candy mold, ice cube tray, or a baking tray, the latter of which is what we used in the recipe below.

The recipe below yields 12 servings.

Time: 3 hours 10 minutes

Serving Size: 1

Prep Time: 10 minutes

Cook Time: 3 hours

Nutritional Facts/Info:

Calories: 137

Carbs: 1.4 grams

Fat: 14.1 grams

Protein: 1.2 grams

Ingredients:

- 4 oz. cream cheese
- 2 tsp. pumpkin spice
- ½ cup pecans
- ½ cup butter
- ½ cup pumpkin purée
- ¼ cup powdered erythritol

Directions:

1. Start by placing your butter and cream cheese in a microwave-safe bowl and allow the two ingredients to soften in the microwave for 30 to 45 seconds, and then mix them together until light yellow and creamy in color and texture.
2. Now, pour the pumpkin purée into the bowl of butter and cheese and combine the ingredients

until a darker shade of yellow is formed and the mixture is creamy in texture.
3. Proceed by stirring the powdered erythritol and pumpkin spice into the same mixture; the color and texture should still be the same as above.
4. Place some parchment or wax paper onto your baking tray before pouring the fully combined mixture onto the parchment paper. Smooth out the top of the mixture with a non-stick spoon. Ensure the mixture is 1 inch thick in height.
5. Sprinkle on your pecans, being sure that they sink just enough into the mixture, before putting the baking tray in the freezer for a maximum time of 3 hours.
6. Once the 3 hours are done, you can remove the baking tray from the freezer and proceed by heating the blade of your knife in hot water, which should make it easier to cut the mold, before cutting the fat bomb mold into 12 even pieces or even smaller pieces if that is what you prefer.

Portobello Mushroom Fries

Portobello Mushroom Fries are the perfect snack to have on the weekend when you just want to enjoy tender fries covered in melted cheese and tasty spices, and you are allowed to substitute the cheese and spices mentioned in the recipe for your own spices and cheese preferences.

Additional notes:

- For added crunch, color, and flavor, you can add chopped scallions or red bell pepper to the recipes. You can add one of these or both on top of the cheese before you melt the cheese in the oven.

The recipe below yields 2 servings of fries and tastes better straight out of the oven; therefore, if you only want to make one serving, then halve the ingredients.

Time: 25 minutes

Serving Size: 1

Prep Time: 15 minutes

Cook Time: 10 minutes

Nutritional Facts/Info:

Calories: 119.5

Carbs: 4.2 grams

Fat: 12.97 grams

Protein: 31.93 grams

Ingredients:

- 2 large Portobello mushroom caps
- 1 large egg
- 1 tbsp. dried chives
- ½ cup shredded Parmesan cheese
- ½ tsp. garlic powder
- ½ tsp. smoked paprika
- ¼ tsp. cayenne pepper
- ¼ cup shredded cheddar cheese

Directions:

- Preheat the oven to 425 degrees Fahrenheit.
- After that, start by washing your mushrooms before placing them on a cutting board.
- Once the mushrooms are on the board, cut them into thick slices; they should resemble the shape of French fries.
- Now, in a small bowl, mix together the Parmesan cheese, cheddar cheese, smoked paprika, dried chives, and cayenne pepper. Ensure that both of the cheese is thinly shredded.
- Set the bowl of cheese and spices aside before lining your baking tray with some and then bring out a shallow dish.
- Whisk your egg together in the shallow dish with garlic powder and another seasoning of

your choice and coat the mushroom slices in the eggy mix. Then lay the coated slices out on the baking tray and put the tray in the oven, allowing the slices to bake for a maximum of 10 minutes.
- Remove the tray from the oven and cover the mushroom fries in the cheese and spice mixture before putting the tray back in the oven for another 5 minutes.
- Once the cheese has melted, you can remove the tray from the oven, dish out the fries, and enjoy right away.

Avocado & Goat Cheese Bites

Avocado & Goat Cheese Bites are a colorful snack that combines the wonderful tastes of avocado, radicchio lettuce, and goat cheese. The snack only takes 15 minutes to make and is ideally low in both carbs and calories.

The recipe below makes 16 little enjoyable bites that are best stored in an airtight container in your fridge, and it should contain the freshness of the ingredients for a maximum of 2 days.

Time: 15 minutes

Serving Size: 1

Prep Time: 15 minutes

Cook Time: N/A

Nutritional Facts/Info:

Calories: 91

Carbs: 0.9 grams

Fat: 7.5 grams

Protein: 4.7 grams

Ingredients:

- 1 large avocado
- 8 oz. goat cheese, softened
- 2 cloves garlic, grated
- 3.9 oz. radicchio lettuce
- 1 tbsp. oregano
- 1 tbsp. rosemary
- 1 tbsp. basil
- 1 tbsp. kosher salt
- 1 tbsp. black pepper

Directions:

1. Start by cutting the stem off the bottom of the radicchio lettuce. Collect 16 fresh medium-sized leaves from the lettuce, and store the

remains in a tightly sealed container for other near-future recipes.
2. Thoroughly wash the leaves, then lay them out on a cutting board or kitchen tray to dry while you grate the garlic cloves, and then put the grated garlic in a medium-sized bowl.
3. Sprinkle the oregano, rosemary, basil, salt, and pepper; mix in the softened goat cheese until the ingredients in the bowl resemble a white chunky paste.
4. Next, you need to cut the large avocado into 16 thick slices, cut each slice in 2, place 2 smaller slices on a radicchio leaf, and scoop 1 tbsp. of the goat cheese mix onto the avocado.
5. Repeat the above process with the other leaves and then you can serve and enjoy.

Chapter 9: Vegetarian Keto Dessert Ideas

Blackberry Pudding

Blackberry Pudding is an amazing after-dinner dish. The dessert is light and fluffy and sweet to the taste. You will seriously enjoy this dish, so we recommend that you do not overindulge.

This recipe yields 2 servings.

Time: 35 minutes

Serving Size: 1

Prep Time: 10 minutes

Cook Time: 25 minutes

Nutritional Facts/Info:

Calories: 459.5

Carbs: 4.91 grams

Fat: 44.04 grams

Protein: 9.1 grams

Ingredients:

- ¼ cup blackberries
- ¼ cup coconut flour
- ¼ tsp. baking powder
- 1 lemon (zested)
- 10 drops liquid Stevia
- 2 tablespoons erythritol
- 2 tbsp. butter
- 2 tbsp. coconut oil
- 2 tbsp. heavy cream
- 2 tsp. lemon juice
- 5 large egg yolks

Directions:

- Turn on the oven and set the temperature to 350 degrees Fahrenheit.
- You will need two small dishes and a spoon to separate the yolks from the egg whites: break the egg inside one bowl, then spoon out the egg yolk and transfer the yolk to the second bowl. Repeat the action with the remaining four eggs.
- You can cover and put away the bowl of egg whites in your fridge, and use them for an egg-white veggie breakfast the next day.

- Whisk the egg yolks together, then add the erythritol and liquid Stevia, and whisk together until fully combined.
- Next, add the lemon juice, the zest of one lemon, heavy cream, coconut oil, and the butter. Stir the ingredients together until mixed.
- Now, add the coconut flour and baking powder to the bowl and mix until fully combined. The mixture is slightly thick and bright yellow in color.
- Add blackberries to the mix before scooping the mixture into two oven-safe small bowls, and bake in the oven for 20 minutes.
- Allow the pudding to cool and it should be slightly liquefied on the inside and the top of the pudding should be brown on the sides.
- Serve and enjoy as is.

Coconut Chip Cookies

Coconut Chip Cookies are a craving-combating kind of cookie. They are not only crunchy and chewy but they are also healthy and keto-friendly. It does not mean you can overindulge, but you sure can enjoy them every now and again.

The recipe below yields 16 cookies.

Time: 35 minutes

Serving Size: 1 cookie

Prep Time: 10 minutes

Cook Time: 25 minutes

Nutritional Facts/Info:

Calories: 192.38

Carbs: 2.17 grams

Fat: 17.44 grams

Protein: 4.67 grams

Ingredients:

- 20 drops liquid Stevia
- 2 large eggs
- 1 cup almond flour
- ½ cup cacao nibs
- ½ cup unsweetened coconut flakes
- ½ almond butter
- ⅓ erythritol
- ¼ cup melted butter
- ¼ tsp. salt
- 1 tsp. vanilla extract

Directions:

1. Turn the oven on and set the temperature to 350 degrees Fahrenheit.
2. Begin by setting out the required ingredients, measuring cups, and a medium bowl for mixing.
3. In a microwaveable cup, melt the butter for 30 seconds in the microwave, and then pour the melted butter into the mixing bowl.
4. Whisk the butter for a second before adding the almond butter, eggs, liquid Stevia, and vanilla extract.
5. Once the wet ingredients are properly combined, the mixture should be coffee brown in color and not too watery.
6. You are going to add, then stir, add, then stir the dry ingredients, one by one. Start with the cacao nibs, then almond flour, coconut flakes, erythritol, and add the salt last. The mixture should be soft, doughy, and brown when properly combined.
7. Now, lay out some wax paper on your baking tray or use a non-stick spray if you do not have wax paper, and use a spoon to scoop out and evenly flatten out 16 cookies on the tray.
8. Bake the cookies for 25 minutes or until the sides begin to brown. Once you take the cookies out of the oven, allow them to cool before serving.

Peanut Butter Balls

Peanut Butter Balls are a quick and simple dessert or snack to make, and it satisfies any cravings you may have. When it comes to storing you can keep these in the fridge.

The recipe yields 15 Coconut Peanut Butter Balls.

Time: 3 hours 10 minutes

Serving Size: 1

Prep Time: 10 minutes

Cook Time: 3 hours

Nutritional Facts/Info:

Calories: 35.13

Carbs: 1.51 grams

Fat: 3.19 grams

Protein: 0.98 grams

Ingredients:

- ½ cup unsweetened shredded coconut
- 2 ½ tsp. powdered erythritol
- 2 tsp. almond flour

- 3 tbsp. creamy peanut butter
- 3 tsp. unsweetened cocoa powder

Directions:

1. Start by whisking the peanut butter in the mixing bowl for 15 to 20 seconds.
2. Then add in the cocoa powder and beat together until smooth and brown in color, and then mix in the erythritol and the almond flour.
3. Once the mixture is combined, it should resemble a browned peanut butter. Now, place the mix in the freezer for 1 hour.
4. The mixture should be firm and you can use a teaspoon to scoop and measure the size of the balls, and then mold them with your hands before dumping them in a bowl of shredded coconut.
5. Place the balls back in the freezer for 1 to 2 hours to set before serving.

Frosty

Absolutely the best dessert idea yet and is totally capable of curing your ice-cream craving, and is not too sweet. The recipe yields four servings. You can store the remains in the freezer, and allow it to sit aside if it happens to be completely frozen.

Time: 50 minutes

Serving Size: 4

Prep Time: 15 minutes

Cook Time: 35 minutes

Nutritional Facts/Info:

Calories: 164

Carbs: 14.1 grams

Fat: 17 grams

Protein: 1.4 grams

Ingredients:

- 2 tbsp. cocoa powder
- 3 tbsp. erythritol
- 1 tsp. vanilla extract
- 1 ½ cup heavy whipping cream
- A pinch of salt

Directions:

- Use a large bowl to whisk together the cream, cocoa, erythritol, vanilla, and salt.

- Dish the mixture into a sealable bag and store in the freezer for 35 minutes.
- The mixture should be just frozen when you pull it out of the freezer, at which point you cut a corner piece of the plastic bag, and squeeze the mixture into a tall glass or bowl.
- Serve and enjoy.

Low-Carb Carrot Cake

Low-Carb Carrot Cake can be keto-friendly if made correctly, but if you do not trust your baking abilities, then substitute the carrot with zucchini instead, which is equally as tasty and twice as satisfying.

Other things to note about the recipe:

- You can use sunflower seed flour instead of almond flour.
- You do not have to use pecans in this recipe.
- Do not replace the sweetener in this recipe with a liquid sweetener.
- Your safest bet with this recipe is to grate the carrot yourself and not use grated carrots from a bag.

The recipe below yields 8 slices that you can store in the fridge for a period of 3 days in a tightly sealed container to ensure the cake does not dry out.

Time: 40 minutes

Serving Size: 1 slice

Prep Time: 15 minutes

Cook Time: 20 minutes

Nutritional Facts/Info:

Calories: 387

Carbs: 4.7 grams

Fat: 35.6 grams

Protein: 9.7 grams

Ingredients:

- 7 tbsp. butter
- 4 large eggs
- 4 oz. cream cheese
- 2 tbsp. cinnamon powder
- 1 tsp. vanilla extract
- 1 tbsp. heavy cream
- 1 tbsp. baking powder
- ¾ cup erythritol
- ½ tsp. ginger powder

- ½ nutmeg powder
- ½ cup pecans
- 1.5 cups almond flour
- 1 large carrot

Directions:

1. Start by turning on your oven to 350 degrees Fahrenheit, getting your baking tray out, and putting wax paper on the baking sheet.
2. Then, in a small bowl, you will make your cream cheese frosting by whisking together the softened 4 oz. of cream cheese, 2 tbsp. of butter, 1 tsp. of vanilla extract, 1 tbsp. of heavy cream, and ¼ cup powdered erythritol until smooth and creamy.
3. Place the bowl of cream cheese frosting in the fridge for later use.
4. Proceed by chopping your pecans into pieces, and then put them aside.
5. Now, in a large bowl, combine the melted remaining 5 tbsp. of butter and the remaining ½ cup of erythritol and whisk these ingredients together until smooth.
6. Whisk in the 4 eggs before stirring in the baking powder, cinnamon, ginger, nutmeg, and vanilla extract.
7. Finally, pour in the chopped pecans, almond flour, and your grated carrot into the same bowl and combine the ingredients until oat-like in color and texture.

8. Pour the mixture into the baking tray lined with wax paper, smooth out with a spoon, and bake in the oven for 20 minutes. (You can test the readiness of the cake by sticking a tooth-pick or fork in the center of the cake; if the tooth-pick or fork comes back clean, then the cake is ready.)
9. Once the cake has been baked, allow the cake to cool for about 10 to 15 minutes, then layer the top of the cake in cream cheese frosting, cut into eight pieces, and serve or store for later enjoyment.

Low-Carb Chia Pudding

Yes, another pudding, but this has to be the most creative dessert recipe yet.

This low-carb dessert could even work as an enjoyable breakfast meal. You could add some strawberries and other keto-friendly fruit like cantaloupe as a topping to really make the recipe your own.

The recipe below yields 3 servings.

Time: 25 minutes

Serving Size: 1 short glass

Prep Time: 25 minutes

Cook Time: N/A

Nutritional Facts/Info:

Calories: 187.07

Carbs: 4.53 grams

Fat: 11.47 grams

Protein: 6.27 grams

Ingredients:

- 2 tsp. unsweetened cocoa powder
- 2 tbsp. monk fruit sweetener
- 1 tsp. vanilla extract
- 1 ½ cups unsweetened almond milk
- ½ cup chia seeds
- 4 strawberries

Directions:

1. First, gather all the above-mentioned ingredients along with any other keto-friendly fruits you want to add to the dessert recipe. (Be sure to check your macros, specifically your intake of carbs for this meal and what you consume the rest of the day to ensure you are not kicked out of ketosis.)

2. In a large bowl, stir together the chia seeds, unsweetened almond milk, monk fruit sweetener, and vanilla extract. Place the bowl in the fridge for 20 minutes.
3. During the 20 minutes, gather your strawberries, cut each strawberry in four, and use a sifter and large spoon to purée the strawberries into a small bowl.
4. Once the 20 minutes have passed, bring out two more other bowls, divide the chia seed mix into three bowls (the two bowls you brought out and the one bowl with the strawberry purée).
5. Pour the strawberry and chia mix evenly into your dessert glasses once you have combined the two recipes.
6. Add unsweetened cocoa powder to the second bowl of chia seed mix and, once you have fully combined the ingredients, pour them evenly into the same three glasses you did the strawberry chia.
7. The last bowl is vanilla and does not need to be combined with anything else, so add that to the glasses, and top the dessert with heavy cream or keto-friendly fruit and enjoy.

Peanut Butter Chocolate Cups

Peanut Butter Chocolate Cups are the treat that curb both your peanut butter and possible chocolate cravings. You can store these for three weeks in the fridge and for 3 months in the freezer. Although, if you are going to store them in the freezer, allow them to 'cool' outside of the freezer for 15 minutes before consumption (to allow for the chocolate to soften a bit and make eating easier).

Additional notes:

- You are going to need cupcake molds.
- You can substitute the peanut butter for keto-friendly seed butter if you wish to avoid nuts.
- Another substitution you can make is to use coconut oil in the place of butter.
- We use sugar-free plain peanut butter but you can use a keto-friendly alternative.
- As for the chocolate, stick to a sugar-free and low-carb chocolate.

The recipe below yields 8 chocolate peanut butter cups.

Time: 50 minutes

Serving Size: 1

Prep Time: 30 minutes

Cook Time: 20 minutes

Nutritional Facts/Info:

Calories: 204.9

Carbs: 3.4 grams

Fat: 19.3 grams

Protein: 4.1 grams

Ingredients:

- 4 oz. low-carb milk chocolate
- ½ tsp. vanilla extract
- ½ cup peanut butter
- ⅓ cup erythritol powder
- ¼ cup butter

Directions:

1. Start by placing your silicone cupcake molds in your cupcake tray.
2. Continue by placing a sauce pan on the stove and set the temperature to a low-medium heat.
3. Scoop the butter into the saucepan and stir until smooth, then stir in the powdered erythritol, peanut butter, and vanilla extract until the mixture is creamy and brown in texture and color.
4. Pour the mixture into the silicone molds and place the cupcake tray in the freezer for 15 minutes.

5. During the 15 minutes, pour some water into a small pot, place the temperature on a medium heat and let the water boil before placing a bowl wide enough to fit over the opening on the pot. Set the temperature to a low heat.
6. Pour your chocolate into the bowl and stir together with a whisk until the chocolate is smooth and creamy, and once the 15 minutes have passed, remove the peanut butter molds from the freezer.
7. Allow the chocolate to cool slightly, as you don't want to melt your peanut butter molds. Once cooled, pour the chocolate out evenly between the 8 molds.
8. Lastly, put the tray back in the freezer for 15 minutes, then remove before carefully removing the peanut butter cups from their molds, and you can enjoy right away and store the rest in a tightly sealed container.

Conclusion

There are three main aspects you learned about in this guide and they are how to:

#1. Effectively Lose Weight on the Ketogenic Diet

The ketogenic diet is a low-carb, high-fat, and moderate-protein diet. When there are no carbs in the body to be burnt for energy, the body defaults to using fat for fuel. When the body has this metabolic reaction, we call it ketosis. However, we do not only lose weight on the ketogenic diet because of what we eat but also from how we choose to eat (our number of meals) and how many calories we choose to consume all together. The key aspects are the high fat and low carb components and how this forces your body to burn both the fat from the food you eat plus your body fat for fuel. A vegetarian ketogenic diet should be always combined with regular exercise and watching your calories.

#2. Adopt Healthier Eating Habits

The ketogenic diet and the vegetarian diet both promote healthy eating habits, the former encourages you to eat fewer carbs and consume more healthy fats, and the latter encourages you to stick to a diet that comprises mostly fruits and vegetables. These diets make you conscious of what foods are around you at all times, therefore, over time you eventually develop healthy eating habits because you are made more aware of what you are putting into your body.

#3. Improve on Vegetarian Recipes

The vegetarian-ketogenic combo diet really allows for creative and fun recipes for you to try out. Think of a vegetarian recipe that isn't keto-friendly and think of a way to make it keto-friendly, then add it to your weekly meal plan.

We truly hope this guide has been helpful to you and that you will be able to implement a vegetarian keto diet effectively in your own life. Remember that everything takes time and patience, and you should remain fully determined and focused, and not let any excuse or worry stand in the way of you making the changes you want to see in your life.

Use our guide as a reference when you get started on the ketogenic diet; we believe that this reference will be effective and that the comprehensive chapters have taught you all you need and have wanted to learn about the vegetarian ketogenic diet.

Introduction to Pescatarian Keto Diet

You might be surprised to learn that the Ketogenic Pescatarian Diet has been around a long time—about 100 years. It was initially developed to help children who were experiencing seizures.

But what exactly is keto? The basic premise of the Ketogenic Pescatarian Diet is to eat low carb and high fat. This is counterintuitive to many of us who have traditionally been taught that fat is bad for us, and we should certainly not eat much of it if we hope to lose weight. The truth is, though, that by eating enough of the correct types of fat, your body will enter a metabolic state known as "nutritional ketosis." It might seem more than a little crazy to think you can lose fat by eating fat, but the scientific basis is sound. Our bodies mainly run on glucose, which is the product of the breakdown of carbohydrates such as rice, grains, pasta, cereals, etc. But when we drastically reduce our carbohydrate intake and add a high amount of fat to our diet, our bodies switch from using carbohydrates as fuel to using fat as fuel, and we are then able to reach ketosis.

Nutritional ketosis allows your body to become a fat-burning machine by turning fat into ketones in the liver. Ketones are a secondary form of energy that our bodies need to function. This backup fuel system allows us to track our metabolism into burning stored fat rather than carbohydrates. These ketones become the primary source of energy for our organs, muscles, and brain to function correctly. Many researchers believe that ketones are a more efficient fuel source than carbohydrates because they burn more slowly, giving your body a more sustainable source of energy.

The Ketogenic Pescatarian Diet is immensely popular thanks to its wide array of benefits. Various studies show that diet can reduce inflammation, increase energy, decrease food cravings (especially for sugar), help clear skin, improve fat burning, slow the effects of aging, and lower the risk of chronic disease. However, one of the most talked-about advantages to living a keto lifestyle is mental clarity.

Neurological inflammation has been linked to reduced cognitive function, as well as depression and anxiety. Just about everyone who has followed the Ketogenic Pescatarian Diet claims to have experienced the benefit of clearer thinking. An overall inflammation most likely causes neurological inflammation that, in turn, affects the brain by increasing focal brain inflammation.

As mentioned, keto was initially used to treat children with epilepsy. Since then, it has proved effective in battling severe illnesses such as diabetes, Parkinson's, and autoimmune diseases, including Hashimoto's. The diet has been shown to increase glutathione, a combination of amino acids that's your body's most potent detoxifier (and something often found lacking in people with autoimmune issues). While in nutritional ketosis, your body will naturally produce more glutathione, which acts as a powerful antioxidant that reduces oxidative stress caused by a poor diet, anxiety, or infection.

Weight loss is also a result of eating a ketogenic diet, and it often happens quickly. Fundamentally, when you starve your body of carbs and sugar, your blood sugar decreases. Your body responds by switching to the alternate form of energy—ketones—and then for as long as you stay in ketosis, your body will continue to burn fat. It is not uncommon for people to lose most of their unwanted pounds in the early stages of keto, while others experience a steady weight loss for as long as they are in ketosis.

Macros, which is short for macronutrients, refers to the three primary nutrients our bodies need to function: protein, fats, and carbohydrates. Your body converts these nutrients into energy for your brain, muscles, and organs. In most diets, macros are tailored toward a person's body type, activity level, and nutritional needs. For example, some foods recommend a 30 percent fat, 35 percent protein, and 35 percent carbohydrate split of daily calories. Pescatarian ketogenic macros, on the other hand, typically target 70 percent fat, 20 percent protein, and 10 percent net carbs, most of those carbs coming from vegetables.

You may have seen the terms "total carbs" and "net carbs" on food labels. "Total carbs" is the tally of all the sugars, fiber, and indigestible starch in a food item. Our bodies need a tissue to be able to excrete waste products efficiently, but because we cannot digest fiber, it does not affect blood sugar levels. "Net carbs" refer to the carbohydrates that can be converted into sugar in our bodies and therefore affect blood sugar levels.

When calculating net carbs, it's essential to ignore sugar alcohols. These are organic compounds found in vegetables, fruit, and many sugar-free products. They have a much lower impact on blood sugar than regular sugars, which is why they are typically subtracted when calculating net carbs. Here's the formula:

Total carbohydrates − fiber − sugar alcohols = net carbs

While you are on the ketogenic diet, you will want to pay attention to the foods you buy to make sure you keep within the 10 percent carbohydrate ratio for your total overall daily calories. The good news is that you don't need to carry around a calculator to track your macros on the keto diet. There are several helpful apps (available for a small monthly fee) that you can customize for individual macro percentages. Some of my favorites are MyFitnessPal, Calorie King, and Carb Manager. You may also find it helpful to keep a food journal, at least until you become accustomed to the diet.

As mentioned, many people associate the keto diet with having to consume a great deal of meat, particularly fatty steak and bacon. Not enough studies have been done to calculate the health risks of such high meat consumption on a long-term basis. Even if you're not a Pescatarian, you may have come to this book because you're curious about the Ketogenic Pescatarian Diet and eager to try it for its multiple benefits, but you are concerned about the diet's overreliance on meat consumption. The good news is that a Pescatarian keto diet is possible and comes with its own set of benefits.

Most Pescatarian s rely heavily on carbohydrates such as beans, rice, pasta, and bread to keep them full. One challenge of following the ketogenic Pescatarian diet, therefore, is figuring out how to replace those carbs with a higher amount of fat and protein. Fortunately, if you're already a plant-based eater, you're likely used to alternative forms of protein such as edamame, tofu, eggs, and some dairy products. Switching from using carbs for fuel to using fat should be reasonably easy for you since you are already comfortable with making substitutions.

People decide to adopt a Ketogenic Pescatarian Diet for different reasons, whether it is to manage their blood sugar better, to lose weight, or even to reduce dependence on certain prescription medications. All of these benefits can come from eating keto. Plant-based diets have some pretty incredible benefits as well, including lowering high blood pressure, keeping cholesterol in check, and reducing overall inflammation that can be caused by animal proteins. So, it only makes sense to combine the Pescatarian and ketogenic diets into one super diet.

Chapter 1: The Basics of the Keto Diet

This will highlight the necessary information needed before starting the ketogenic diet. Understanding the main principles of keto, how it works, and steps to take before starting will ensure a more successful experience! The keto diet offers numerous benefits that will also be outlined in this.

What Is Keto?

The ketogenic weight loss plan, or keto for short, is a diet that makes a specialty of ingesting little to no carbs, however excessive quantities of fat.
The result of eating in such a manner forces the frame right into a metabolic state called ketosis. During ketosis, the structure makes use of fat as energy due to the absence of carbs. Typically, glucose is the primary supply of energy. Glucose is derived from carbs.

The fats consumed through food are used as energy, but ketosis is also successful in using fat stores in the body as well. This process is compelling for those looking to lose high amounts of body fat. The process starts in the liver, where the body converts fat into ketones. Ketones are what replace or act like glucose while you follow the keto diet. Ketones are always present when in ketosis. In simple terms, when the body is in ketosis, ketones are being used as energy instead of glucose.

Although there are many different keto diet versions, the standard keto diet or SKD is the most popular. Other versions are supervised by health professionals or used by athletes. All versions of the keto diet rely on the same concepts but may alter carbohydrate levels based on unique circumstances. An SKD diet is classified as 75% fat, 20% protein, and only 5% carbs (Freeman, Kossoff, & Hartman, 2007). Because the Keto diet has strict macronutrient intake, many foods are eliminated. However, much of the keto diet's success comes from consuming an average number of calories. So, the keto diet does not restrict calories but does mostly limit the type of foods that can be eaten. Many diets fail because the temptations of overeating are too high. With the keto diet, you'll never go hungry, and many modifications can be made so the same foods can be enjoyed.

What Are the Benefits of Keto?

One of the main reasons many start the keto diet is to lose weight. The Ketogenic Pescatarian Diet has become well known and popular among many due to its ability to shed a large number of pounds, fast. A study found that those on the keto diet lost 2.2 times more weight than those on a calorie-restricted, low-fat diet (Brehm et al., 2003). As mentioned, part of the success of the keto diet is its no restrictiveness in terms of calories. Feeling full and satisfied is allowed and also encouraged. Eating lots of healthy fats provides a sense of comfort, but it also helps keep energy levels up. On calorie-restricting diets, lethargic and binge-eats are common because the body always feels like it's missing something. The keto diet allows fat loss without restricting or controlling food, making the menu more suitable for everyday life. Food elimination is essential, while restricting calories is not.

Other reasons the keto diet is successful for weight loss has to do with hormones. Leptin and ghrelin, known as the hunger hormones, see a positive change while on the keto diet. Leptin is a hormone made by fat cells that decreases appetite, while ghrelin is the opposite (ghrelin will increase appetite). Both play a crucial role in weight management. Both hormones must maintain a healthy balance, so the brain knows when to stop eating, and your body feels satisfied sooner. Diets that are high in sugar and carbs may trigger leptin resistance, which hinders the brain from feeling full. Leptin resistance is a problem because the brain doesn't know when to stop eating or see when the body is starving. Cloudy signals lead to overeating and a false sense of hunger. According to Perfect Keto (2019), the keto diet decreases ghrelin levels, reduces hunger, and regulates leptin. A controlled appetite, increased satiety and fat burning, higher leptin sensitivity, and the prevention of insulin resistance are the scientific reasons the keto diet is excellent for weight loss.

The keto food plan is frequently advocated for those suffering from type diabetes and for prediabetics. Diabetes is diagnosed as adjustments within the metabolism, high blood sugar, and impaired insulin function. Insulin is a hormone made within the pancreas regulating blood sugar stages from getting too excessive or low. Insulin can be the central aspect of weight gain or excess fat storage. When the frame doesn't respond to insulin, extra is produced. This can be brought about by sugar, carbs, an unhealthy lifestyle, or lack of exercise. However, I have a look at located that the keto weight-reduction plan progressed insulin sensitivity by way of 75% (Boden et al., 2005)! The examination suggests that many had been capable of forestalling the usage of all diabetes medications. (However, before you anticipate your prescription, get permitted from your physician first!) The weight loss plan's capacity to enhance insulin sensitivity has proven helpful for type two diabetes and prediabetic situations.

Other conditions have additionally shown advantageous modifications when uncovered to a ketogenic lifestyle. Those situations include but aren't restricted to coronary heart disease, positive cancers, Alzheimer's disease, epilepsy, Parkinson's disease, polycystic ovary syndrome, mind injuries, and acne (Mawer, 2020).

In everyday life, the keto diet offers increased energy and focus. Many report feelings of mental clarity, improved concentration, and higher energy levels while on the keto diet. Fortunately, there is no placebo effect when it comes to these feelings because all three are backed by science. The simple explanation is that ketones are a better source of energy than glucose, as ketones can carry more energy per unit when combined with oxygen than glucose (Fan, 2013). This means that when oxygen is breathed in, a more significant response occurs when the oxygen reaches a ketone than glucose. This stimulates and creates a more substantial response from the brain and translates into various mental benefits. From a cellular perspective, the mitochondria in brain cells receive more oxygen when ketones are present, which produces more brain activity.

In summary, the keto diet offers many health benefits and has shown improvements in certain diseases or medical conditions. Whether starting the diet to lose weight or manage a condition, rest assured there are benefits for all.

Starting a new diet or lifestyle can be challenging. However, the keto diet is one of the easiest to implement. With that being said, there are a few steps to take beforehand to maximize success.

The first step is to prepare for the changes coming mentally. It's essential to make and visualize the journey ahead psychologically. For many, writing down goals and aspirations proves helpful. Avoiding foods or unhealthy habits you once enjoyed will be even more complicated if the end goals are not clear. During this step, write down all of the reasons a change is necessary. After reading about the benefits, be sure to include which apply most and are the most intriguing. If the main goal is to lose weight, write down all the desired outcomes, and how you will feel once that goal is achieved.

Once a list has been prepared, put it in a safe place to reference when times get hard. It's also recommended to keep a weekly blog. It will be easier to make adjustments for quicker results, but your progress can be tracked. Seeing the positive changes from week to week is encouraging! Not all changes will be physical, so a short entry detailing other positive changes is necessary. Staying in tune with goals weekly and monitoring the positive changes will help you to keep going!

Related to the above, before you start keto, it is also recommended to go for a check-up with your health care provider and run some simple blood work for cholesterol, creatinine, a complete blood count, your fasting blood glucose, and hemoglobin A1c (Bourdua-Roy et al., n.d.). These results are essential as low-carb diets can have adverse indications, and these can only be seen when you visit the lab and get the results. Ideally, get your types of blood tested every three months.

The second step is to consider telling a close friend or partner all the goals you wish to achieve. An accountability partner may be helpful but isn't necessary if you feel uncomfortable. Talking with an accountability partner or someone in a similar situation can increase motivation. Sharing frustrations or goals is healthy for mental health and creates a release that subdues stress.

Lifestyle changes aren't always easy, and sharing wins and defeats can make the journey easier. If you're comfortable sharing your lifestyle change, it may be easier to stick to the keto guidelines and avoid temptations in social settings. However, not all situations will prompt questions from others, and most of the time, many won't notice the skipped treat or breadstick. Step one will be of extra benefit if you prefer to keep your changes private.

The third step to take before starting the keto diet is cleaning out the pantry or rearranging. If you're living with others, it might not be possible to get rid of treats or temptations. Consider keeping your food in a unique location where other people's diet isn't visible. For example, your pantry can be created and does not have to be in a traditional "pantry" location. In the refrigerator, keep your food organized and in one place. This will help prevent the urge to cheat or binge. The keto diet is safe and healthy for most, and the entire household/family can participate. For example, chips, bread, treats, and more can still be enjoyed with some modifications. Replace unhealthy foods with keto-approved foods. If you're living alone or making the lifestyle change with your partner, donate the unhealthy foods and get them out of sight! If you're able, control what foods are in the house, so fewer temptations are possible.

By taking these three steps, your chances of a successful keto diet will increase. Staying focused and persistent will yield results! Don't forget to track your progress and make adjustments as necessary.

Chapter 2: Why Choose the Keto Lifestyle?

There are many blessings to the ketogenic weight loss plan, including increased energy, weight loss, and both the remedy and prevention of many diseases. In this, we will discuss a number of the most commonplace motives to select the ketogenic eating regimen and the health-promoting qualities it could provide.

Weight Loss

While science has shown that BMI has little merit and you can be both fat and healthy, and there is no shame in being fat and proud even if you are unhealthy, there is still much scientific backing showing that having a higher body fat percentage increases your risk of disease. Many people may try crash diets to lower their weight, but years of these diets take a toll on your health and reduce your metabolism and make it more challenging to lose weight over time. You often even gain the weight back soon after quitting the diet.

Thankfully, the Ketogenic Pescatarian Diet is not a fad diet; it's been proven to be healthy, and it supports maintainable weight loss. Rather than starving your body of calories and nutrients, you can provide it with ample energy, vitamins, and minerals while enjoying a variety of natural and delicious meals.

When you are on a standard high-carbohydrate diet, the constant assault of carbohydrates on your body causes an insulin and blood sugar response. It prevents your body from burning off the digested fat and body fat. Yet when you are on a low-carbohydrate and high-fat diet, your body is burning off fat by default. Not only will it burn off the fat you consume, but it will also burn off your body fat and increase your metabolism, helping you to lose weight.

The rate of your weight loss can be customized, depending on how much of a caloric deficit you are eating. It is unhealthy to lose more than two to three pounds a week, so if after the first two weeks of the Ketogenic Pescatarian Diet, you are losing more than this, then adjust your caloric deficit so that you are losing weight at a slightly slower pace. Though you may lose quite a bit the first couple of weeks in water weight, this should not concern you.

Need to gain weight, you can accomplish that on the Ketogenic Pescatarian Diet by merely adjusting your caloric intake. Some people may consume twelve-hundred calories a day; others may consume sixteen-hundred, while others are two-thousand. It all depends on the needs of your body, your doctor's recommendations, and whether or not you have an eating disorder.

Lower Your Cholesterol

We are used to hearing about how bad fats are for us, causing disease, and clog our arteries. Since the war on fat in the 1990s and early 2000s, people have been afraid of fat, even from health sources. While there was a little truth to this, certain fats, such as trans fats, are bad for you, and there are many healthy fats. Yet fats such as those found in avocados, olives, sesame seeds, coconut, and nuts have been found to have fantastic health benefits and weight loss promoting qualities. The Ketogenic Pescatarian Diet and these healthy sources of fats have been shown to lower dangerous cholesterol, increase healthy cholesterol, and reduce the risk of developing cardiovascular diseases.

If you have heard about the Ketogenic Pescatarian Diet raising cholesterol, it was most likely a misunderstanding, as this has never been shown to be true. On the contrary, multiple studies have shown the cholesterol-lowering properties of the ketogenic diet.

The good cholesterol, which the Ketogenic Pescatarian Diet does raise, is necessary to lower bad cholesterol. This type of cholesterol boosts vitamin D absorption, manages hormones, and aids in the digestion of food. Good cholesterol, known as HDL, is entirely harmless and promotes increased health.

There are two types of dangerous cholesterol, not one. These are LDL and the lesser-known VLDL. These cause a buildup of plaque in the arteries and increase the risk of a heart attack. On one study of the ketogenic diet, sixty-six obese patients who experienced high cholesterol went on the Ketogenic Pescatarian Diet and were able to lose weight, increase good cholesterol, lower bad cholesterol, as well as blood glucose and triglycerides. The study was deemed successful and that the Ketogenic Pescatarian Diet was shown to be a valuable treatment against high cholesterol and heart disease.

Reduce Aging

The mitochondrial cells can utilize amino acids, fatty acids, and glucose for fuel. These cells are required to produce ninety percent of the energy our body needs, and we are unable to survive without them. If these cells are not thriving, then neither can we.

While incredibly powerful and necessary, sometimes while converting fuel into energy for our cells, electrons can escape. This process will cause dangerous free radicals to form, and worse yet, these are the most dangerous type of free radicals, known as reactive oxygen species.

While this process is a natural part of aging and happens without most people being aware, it does cause cellular damage and degradation. Thankfully, the Ketogenic Pescatarian Diet can fight against this process by increasing the number of mitochondrial cells, increasing the cell's ability to convert energy efficiently. It contains many powerful antioxidants that neutralize and remove these free radicals. This not only slows down the aging of your skin but your entire body and mind.

The Ketogenic Pescatarian Diet has impressive benefits for treating seizures, both those caused by epilepsy and those that are not. The Ketogenic Pescatarian Diet was created nearly one-hundred years ago to treat epilepsy before anticonvulsants were created. While the Ketogenic Pescatarian Diet declined with the discovery of anticonvulsant drugs, it made a resurgence once people realized that drugs are ineffective in many people. While the Ketogenic Pescatarian Diet alone is not for everyone with uncontrolled epilepsy, it has been shown to reduce seizures in many cases significantly. This is especially great as anticonvulsants have a high rate of side effects, including drowsiness, sleepiness, and mental fatigue. These symptoms get in the way of life and even many people's jobs, making it hard to stay on the anticonvulsants, also if needed. Thankfully, the Ketogenic Pescatarian Diet provides people with more options.

There have been countless studies demonstrating the success of treating seizures and epilepsy with the ketogenic diet. In one study that took place at Trinity College between 2001 and 2006, there were one-hundred and forty-five participants. All of these participants were resistant to drug therapy in the past. Out of these patients, seven percent experienced a reduction of more than ninety percent in seizure activity. Thirty-eight percent of the people experienced an improvement of over fifty percent reduction in seizure activity.

While for most people on the ketogenic diet, the body will provide enough ketones for their needs, those with neurological and neurodegenerative diseases may want to boost their ketones, even more, to protect their brains from potential damage caused by the illness. In this case, MCT oil (medium-chain triglycerides) and exogenous ketones have been found to provide benefits and further reduce seizure activity. While some children who have sensitive stomachs may not be able to handle the ketogenic diet, while not as effective, MCT and exogenous ketones along may provide a small amount of benefit. This is because both of these products increase the number of ketones available to protect the brain; therefore, preventing seizures.

While most of our cells can use ketones as a fuel source rather than glucose, this is not true of cancer and tumor cells. This means that when you are on the ketogenic diet, the meager amount of glucose in your body and the production of ketones can starve cancer and tumor cells of energy to grow. Some studies have shown that within a few days of beginning the ketogenic diet, tumor cells, whether cancerous or not, have been shown to start shrinking. It has also been shown to halt tumor growth, improve symptoms, and increase the effectiveness of chemotherapy. All of these benefits from the Ketogenic Pescatarian Diet for treating cancer are reversed if the person discontinues the ketogenic diet.

Age-related diseases have dramatically increased over the years, and Alzheimer's is the most common and debilitating of these diseases. Startling, there are nearly forty-four million people worldwide who have either Alzheimer's disease or related dementia, and out of these people, Alzheimer's Disease International estimates that one in four will be diagnosed.

Not only is this disease severe on the person diagnosed, but on the family as well. It takes a toll on the family's emotions, time, and finances, but in 2016, 15.9 million family members provided care at an estimated 18.2 billable hours, which is 240 billion dollars.

The worst news is that Alzheimer's disease is the sixth leading cause of death in the United States, and typical life expectancy after diagnosis is only four to eight years. Startlingly, between the years of 2000 and 2014, there was an eighty-nine percent increase in deaths from Alzheimer's disease, and it is estimated that between 2017 and 2025, there will be a 14% increase in the condition.

This disease causes the neurons in the brain to develop insulin resistance, making it difficult for them to absorb glucose and therefore stave for fuel. Thankfully, not only do ketones act as a non-glucose fuel source for these cells, but the diet has also been shown to decrease insulin resistance. This will provide the cells with ketones for fuel, but by treating the insulin resistance, they will better be able to absorb the glucose that is offered to them through the gluconeogenesis process.

One study was conducted on twenty adult participants who lived with either Alzheimer's or other cognitive impairment diseases. In this study, the participants were given either an MCT oil drink, which increases ketone levels or a placebo. Within ninety minutes of drinking the MCT drink, people's ketones increased significantly, and they displayed significant improvements in symptoms, whereas the placebo-control group did not improve.

In another study, a patient with Alzheimer's disease went on a treatment protocol with coconut oil and MCT oil for twenty months. The patient experienced significant improvement and success. They improved fourteen points on the scale of Activities of Daily Living and six points on the Alzheimer's Disease

Assessment Scale-Cognitive. The patient experienced a remarkable improvement in mood, word-finding, recalling events, social participation, tremors, and gait during this time. MRI scans conducted throughout the test period displayed that his brain experienced no decline during the twenty-month treatment period.

A study that compared the effects of high-carbohydrate diets and low-carbohydrate diets on senior adults found that the participants on a low-carbohydrate diet showed improved functioning. These patients experienced a loss in fat around the abdomen and weight loss, as well as enhanced fasting insulin, memory performance, and fasting glucose. This improvement was concluded to be the result of increased ketones from the diet.

Chapter 3: Who is a Pescatarian?

A pescatarian is someone that includes fish to their diet but avoids meat and other poultry. The term was coined in the early 1990s with a combination of two words, 'Pesce,' which means fish, and 'vegetarian.' In summary, a pescatarian is anyone who follows the vegetarian diet, but also includes fish and other seafood to his or her diet. The menu is mainly made up of plant-based foods like legumes, healthy fats, nuts, whole grains, and produce, with seafood being the primary protein source.

It may interest you to know that several pescatarians eat eggs and dairy too. In the same way that we have several versions of the vegetarian diet, we also have several versions of the pescatarian diet. One can eat a diet free of meat but packed with plenty of junk foods, processed starches, and fish sticks instead of a healthier diet.

What do Pescatarians Eat?

- Peanuts and seeds, nuts and nut butter
- Whole grains and grain products
- Vegetables
- Fruits
- Seeds including flaxseeds, chia, and hemp
- Legumes including lentils, hummus, tofu and beans
- Dairy including cheese, milk, and yogurt
- Shellfish and fish
- Eggs
- What not to Eat
- Pork
- Turkey
- Chicken
- Beef
- Lamb
- Wild game

What Did a Pescatarian Eat?

Pesce means "fish" in Italian, so it's easy to conclude that a pescatarian is a vegetarian who eats fish. But is it that simple? Well, sort of. To make sure we're clear and not missing any of the incredible food groups available in the pescatarian lifestyle, here's an overview of the foods pescatarians eat.

Beans, lentils, and legumes. This category also includes soy products like edamame, tofu, and tempeh. And don't forget chickpeas, which make delectable hummus.

Eggs. Pescatarians differ on eggs—some choose to eat them, some omit them. It's up to you.

Dairy products. As with eggs, some pescatarians eat milk, cheese, yogurt, kefir, and other dairy products, whereas others avoid these foods.

Fruits.

Nuts and seeds. These can be used in a medley of ways to add an abundance of exciting and intriguing flavors and textures to your meals and snacks.

Seafood. Any fish or shellfish that comes from a river, lake, bay, or ocean is fair for a pescatarian.

Vegetables. There's no chance of boredom with the full range of colors, textures, and flavors available from plants!

Whole grains. When paired with other plant-based foods, whole grains like barley, rice, oats, and bread can help create complete proteins, which are essential for people following a mostly plant-based diet.

What Doesn't a Pescatarian Eat?

Though it may go without saying, here's a look at what you'll be leaving off the grocery list when you convert to a pescatarian lifestyle:

Organ meat. Avoid all organ meats and offal—including liver, tongue, sweetbreads, tripe, and chitterlings.

Red meat. Pescatarians avoid all meats that come from mammals and are red in their raw state (beef, lamb, pork, veal, venison, etc.).

Wild game. Although less popular than red meat and white meat, game meats—including pheasant, rabbit, venison, and wild boar—won't make an appearance on a pescatarian's plate.

White meat. Poultry, such as chicken, duck, goose, and turkey, are also off-limits.

Reasons to Change Your Lifestyle

Perhaps you've been an omnivore and are now eliminating meat and poultry from your diet. Or maybe you were a vegetarian and are now reintroducing fish. Here are just a few reasons for choosing a pescatarian lifestyle.

Additional health benefits. Eating less red meat has been shown to lower the risks of developing high blood pressure, heart disease, and cancer. As a pescatarian, you'll consume less saturated fat and experience the benefits of healthy fats found in plant-based food sources and heart-healthy omega-3 fatty acids found in fish, such as salmon and mackerel.

Environmental concerns. Omitting meat from your diet may also be a way to reduce your carbon footprint due to the abundance of natural resources it takes to raise land animals.

Variety. If you've been a vegetarian, adding fish to your diet means more variety in flavor and more sources of essential nutrients, like iron, vitamin B12, and protein.

Weight loss. Omitting red meat, poultry, wild game, and organ meat from your diet means you'll likely be eating a higher amount of nutrient-dense and low-calorie plant-based foods than before, which are generally also lower in calories. Plus, enjoying a variety of seafood will help keep the process from feeling too restrictive.

Reasons to Follow a Pescatarian Diet

Several people follow the pescatarian diet for different reasons. Some of these reasons are:

Health benefits

Research has proven that plant-based diets have several advantages, including lowering the risk of obesity and chronic diseases like diabetes and heart disease. Research also shows that you can get these protective benefits from following the pescatarian diet.

One study proved that women who followed the pescatarian diet gained 2.5 fewer pounds than women who had meat in their food. Also, people who changed their diet to plant-based gained the least amount of weight. This means that reducing your consumption of meat and poultry may be beneficial to your health regardless of your current eating patterns.

Another study concluded that people on a pescatarian diet had reduced the risk of developing diabetes at 4.8 percent compared to omnivores at 7.6 percent.

Also, one study looked at people who were pescatarian or rarely ate meat. It discovered that these people had a 22 percent lower risk of dying from heart diseases than people who eat meat regularly.

Environmental concerns

United Nations quoted that raising livestock contributes to 15 percent of all human-made carbon emissions. While producing fish and other seafood generates lower carbon than any animal meat or cheese.

One study conducted in 2014 calculated that fish eaters' diets caused 46 percent less greenhouse gas emissions than that of people who consumed at least one serving of meat each day.

Ethical reasons

Some people may choose to be vegetarians for ethical reasons, and the same applies to pescatarians. Some ethical reasons for which people may prefer to avoid meat in their diet include:

Inhumane factory practices: they are not in support of factory farms that raise livestock in harsh and inhumane conditions.

Opposing slaughter: they do not support the killing of animals for food.

Humanitarian reasons: they believe producing grain to feed to animals is a waste of resources and land, considering the world's level of hunger.

Poor labor conditions: they do not want to be a part of factory farms that poorly treat their workers.

The Health Benefits of a Pescatarian Lifestyle

The way you feed your body can have a significant impact on your overall health. If you stick to a pescatarian eating plan, you will get all the benefits of a plant-based diet with the additional protein and nutrients of seafood. Plus, you'll eliminate the risks associated with eating meat. Here's just a taste of the benefits you could experience.

Brain health. We all want healthy brains. Studies suggest eating fish may support this. A 2016 study showed that eating at least three servings of fish per week while you're pregnant could benefit your offspring's brain. Research also shows that eating fish can lower the risk of developing Alzheimer's disease.

Heart health. Opting for a pescatarian diet can be a way to nourish your heart. Oily fish, such as mackerel and salmon, are rich in omega-3 fatty acids, which have been shown to reduce the risk of fatal heart attacks and congestive heart failure. And studies have shown that people who follow a plant-based diet are less likely to develop coronary heart disease.

Inflammation. Inflammation is associated with some diseases, and many of the foods in a pescatarian diet star in an anti-inflammatory diet, especially fatty fish, which are rich in omega-3 fats.

Minimizing cancer risk, limiting your intake of red meats and processed meats can reduce your risk of developing certain cancers.

Weight loss. As mentioned earlier, those who follow a pescatarian diet can maintain or lose weight because of the lower calories and higher nutrient density of the foods most frequently eaten in this lifestyle.

Benefits of Adding Fish to a Diet

You will enjoy several benefits when you add fish to the vegetarian diet. Several people are worried that avoiding animal flesh or eliminating animal products could cause a low intake of certain vital nutrients. For instance, it is tough to get protein, calcium, zinc, and vitamin B12 on a vegan diet. When you add seafood like mollusks, crustaceans, and fish to the vegetarian diet, you will begin to enjoy your diet's vital nutrients and varieties.

Get more omega-3s

The better manner to get omega-three fatty acids is by ingesting fish. Some plant-based foods like flaxseed walnuts contain alpha-linolenic acid, which is a type of omega-3 fat. But it is not easy for the body to convert this type of acid to docosahexaenoic acid DHA and eicosapentaenoic acid (EPA). EPA and DHA have more benefits that are helpful to the heart, brain, and mood. Oily fish like sardines and salmon contain both DHA and EPA.

Boost your protein intake

Every person needs a daily intake of about 0.8g of protein per 2.2 pounds of body weight to stay healthy. So, a person who weighs 150 pounds needs to eat a minimum of 54 grams of protein daily. It can be tough to achieve a high protein diet with just plant-based foods, particularly if you do not want extra fat or carbs with your protein. An excellent source of lean protein is fish and other seafood, as it gives your body the protein needed for the body to perform optimally.

Seafood has other nutrients

Apart from protein and omega-3s, seafood is rich in several other nutrients. For example, oysters have a high content of vitamin B12, selenium, and zinc. One oyster gives 55 percent of the RDI for selenium and zinc, as well as 133 percent of the RDI for vitamin B12.

Mussel is another seafood with high contents of selenium, manganese, vitamin B12, and other B vitamins.

Whitefish varieties like flounder and cod do not have many omega-3 fats but provide extremely lean protein. For instance, 3 ounces of cod produces less than a gram of fat and 19 grams of protein. Cod is an excellent choice for people who need niacin, phosphorus, selenium, vitamins B6 and vitamins B12

Gives you more options

The vegetarian diet can be limiting at times, especially when eating out at restaurants. If you eat food to stay healthy, then being a pescatarian offers you more meal options. And fish makes a good option as you can prepare it in several ways; grill, bake or sauté.

Chapter 4: The Pescatarian Diet

To get commenced on our pescatarian weight loss program journey, we want to learn more about it. Pesce is Italian for "fish." A pescatarian food plan is much like a Mediterranean weight loss program, or to a vegetarian food regimen with the addition of fish and seafood. This eating fashion emphasizes minimally processed components and whole-food resources for carbohydrates, protein, and fat. Here are some of the other defining capabilities of this style of eating:

Living in Seattle—home of the famous Pike Place Market fish throwers and many Alaskan fisherpersons and seafood processors—I've always been lucky to have access to incredible seafood. Perhaps that, along with growing up in a Norwegian American family, has contributed to my love of seafood. I hope to share that enthusiasm with you in the that follow. Being a pescatarian may feel restrictive because you are no longer eating red meat or poultry, but I promise you won't feel deprived. Changing your lifestyle also comes with a learning curve. I am excited to share with you the tips and tricks I've gathered from personal experience to help you in your journey to becoming—and staying—a pescatarian.

The 5 Major Principles of The Pescatarian Diet

If you're new to a pescatarian lifestyle, there are several vital components to remember. Although there are many variety and flexibility in this style of eating, some of the most common features are listed below.

Fish and Seafood as Primary Animal Proteins: A pescatarian diet includes fresh and saltwater fish, shellfish, and crustaceans. You won't see ingredients such as beef, pork, poultry, wild game, or other meats.

The Ability to Include Eggs and Dairy: Many pescatarians choose to include eggs and dairy as protein sources. However, some prefer to rely solely on fish and seafood for animal protein. The best part about the pescatarian diet is that the choice is up to you.

Plant-Forward Focus: Many people gravitate toward plant-based eating for health or environmental concerns. A pescatarian diet is similar in that regard and can offer a realistic compromise for people who don't want to go entirely vegetarian.

Lots of Fruits and Vegetables: A pescatarian diet encourages a high intake of fruits and vegetables. These are nutrient-rich ingredients that provide many essential vitamins and minerals and beneficial antioxidants and phytochemicals for health.

Whole Grains and Fiber-Rich Foods: A pescatarian diet is not meant to be a low-carbohydrate diet. It includes carbohydrates from whole grains and other starchy or fiber-rich foods such as potatoes, legumes, and ancient grains.

10 Common Questions About a Pescatarian Diet

It's not unusual to have questions or concerns about adding more fish to your diet. I hope you could read below to learn some of the most common questions I hear as a dietitian.

Will a pescatarian diet help me lose weight?

While there are many ways a pescatarian diet can help you improve health, it is not a weight-loss diet. Weight is not a controllable behavior. We can, however, support good health by eating balanced, nourishing meals. Adopting a pescatarian diet as part of your lifestyle may lead to improvements in health, including some potential weight loss, but weight loss is not guaranteed or our primary goal.

Can I substitute other proteins instead of seafood?

Although a right pescatarian diet doesn't include beef, poultry, pork, or other meats, many families enjoy these foods regardless. This book was written to help you adopt the diet, but if you want to swap out seafood for other animal proteins every once in a while, that is okay. It would be best if you did not eat seafood every day

Should I eat seafood every day?

No. The current recommendation for adults is two to three servings per week (totaling eight to 12 ounces). A pescatarian diet does not require you to include seafood at every meal; in fact, most of your meals could be plant-based.

Is a pescatarian diet safe?

A pescatarian diet is safe for most people, so long as you're aware of which fish contain high levels of mercury. Generally, the higher the fish appears on the food chain, the higher the mercury content. Some of the highest-mercury fish include swordfish, shark, king mackerel, and tilefish. Additionally, pregnant women should avoid more than six ounces of albacore (white) tuna. Pregnant women should also avoid raw fish to reduce the risk of foodborne illness.

Do I have to include eggs or dairy?

Many people who identify as pescatarians include eggs and dairy, but it is a personal choice. There are limitations for someone with lactose intolerance or an allergy to eggs or dairy. In those cases, many alternative products can be used in recipes as a replacement, such as a nut or coconut kinds of milk.

Can I get enough protein on a pescatarian diet?

Yes. Most adults in the United States are easily able to meet the recommended amounts of protein each day. Because a pescatarian diet includes protein from fish and seafood, plant-based protein from various sources, and the option to add eggs and dairy products, there are few concerns about protein intake for those following the diet.

Will I be able to afford the ingredients needed to make these recipes or follow the meal plan?

These recipes include affordable options that are easy to find in most grocery stores. Some types of seafood can be quite expensive, but these recipes are built around fresh or frozen fillets of commonly available fish or canned options for tuna and salmon. There are also tips included for ingredient substitutions if you are unable to find or purchase ingredients called for in a recipe. And because a pescatarian diet doesn't require seafood in every meal, you can further stretch your grocery budget by relying on plant-based meals when you choose to skip seafood.

How long will I have to spend cooking?

Many of the recipes can be made in 30 minutes or less and are labeled as such. If you have even less time, look for the Quick Prep label for meals that require little or no active cooking and take 10 minutes or less to prepare. Some meals, such as slow cooker meals and recipes that need time to chill or freeze, may take longer overall, but the active preparation time will not belong.

How can I make a pescatarian diet more family-friendly?

Introducing any new foods to family meals can be challenging. However, these recipes feature familiar flavors and can be easily modified to fit your family's tastes. Seafood is safe to introduce to infants 6 to 12 months of age, but if you have concerns about food allergies or your child is prone to them, please consult with your pediatrician and dietitian first. As for serving family-friendly pescatarian meals, you can plate ingredients separately, use spices and seasonings more sparingly, or offer dipping sauces or other condiments to appeal to younger children's tastes. For more information on family meals, I recommend resources by Ellyn Satter, including her Division of Responsibilities model of family feeding.

Will a pescatarian diet harm the environment?

If you are conscious about selecting a variety of sustainably caught or farmed seafood, the inclusion of seafood to your diet should not negatively impact the environment. See the on Eco-friendly Fish for more information to guide your decisions.

Chapter 5: Preparing your Pescatarian Kitchen

As a dietitian, one of my favorite catchphrases is "Proper planning provides for peak performance!" While it may be hard to say that five times fast, it couldn't be more accurate than when developing healthy eating habits, like adopting the pescatarian diet.

Without preparation, it's easy to make excuses. Think about it—how many times have you said something like "I don't have beans [or insert any pantry item], so I can't make the bean tacos [or any recipe] I planned. I'll just order takeout instead." One missed dinner turns into two, which turns into several. You forget to restock your pantry, and over time you begin to feel the effects of too much takeout. You're lethargic, bloated from excess salt, and even pack on a few unwanted pounds.

Instead, be prepared for success on the pescatarian diet: stock your pantry, take inventory, and get organized. This way, you'll feel confident in what you're doing. Having a well-stocked kitchen and pantry helps eliminate common obstacles and improves your organization. Frequently used ingredients will be available, you'll cut trips to the supermarket in half, and you'll save time and money. Even more, studies show that being organized can help improve your healthy eating habits and boost your energy, so let's get started.

Stocking the Essentials

Setting a good foundation in your kitchen will help spur your success in adopting the pescatarian lifestyle. First, get prepared. Read this to learn about the essentials for optimal success. Second, take inventory of your current pantry, refrigerator, and freezer. You may have more than you think! Surveying your list will help you save money by avoiding duplicate purchases. This is also an excellent time to toss expired pantry items (or those with too much freezer burn). Organize your pantry using the "first in, first out" system to prevent waste in the future. Place items with a sooner expiration date closer to the front and those with a later date behind them. Next, eliminate what you don't need or use. Donate these items to a local food pantry. Finally, stock up to save time later. Head to the store to restock your pantry, refrigerator, and freezer with the necessities to succeed on a pescatarian plan.

The Pantry

Canned beans: Canned beans are among the most flexible and inexpensive plant-based proteins to stock in your pantry. Full of fiber, too, canned beans can be used in salads, soups, snacks, main dishes, and even desserts (you must try the [Blender Black Bean Brownies](#)).

Canned salmon: As an inexpensive alternative to fresh-caught salmon, canned salmon is packed with protein, omega-3 fatty acids, and even calcium (if it contains bones). For a fraction of the price, you can always eat the pescatarian way if you have canned salmon (and other fish, like sardines and tuna).

These tiny chia seeds are a nutritious superstar and versatile in the kitchen. Sprinkle them on any dish for an extra nutrient boost as they contain a balance of healthy fats, plant-based protein, and fiber. Plus, when added to liquid, chia seeds gel, absorbing up to nine times their weight in liquid and creating a pudding-like texture.

Diced canned tomatoes: Did you know that US-grown canned tomatoes go from farm to can within hours? This locks in their nutrients, including lycopene, vitamins C and E, and potassium, so you get the most out of this seasonal fruit. Plus, canned tomatoes contain more of the antioxidant lycopene than fresh vegetables, which helps reduce inflammation and ward off chronic diseases.

Dry whole-grains (farro, buckwheat, bulgur, quinoa, etc.): Whole-grains are a staple on the pescatarian diet because they're high in fiber, vitamins, and minerals. Replacing refined white grains with whole-grains will boost your heart health, improve blood sugar control, and more. There are more than 20 types of whole-grains to choose from, so have fun experimenting over time.

Quality oils: Not all oils are created equally. Opt for pure heart-healthy oils rich in monounsaturated fats, like olive oil and avocado oil. Avocado oil is the preferred option for higher cooking temperatures because of its higher smoke point, while olive oil is used in dressings and marinades; however, both can safely be used interchangeably.

Rolled oats: A deliciously nutritious breakfast staple, multipurpose oats are rich in fiber, B vitamins, magnesium, iron, and more, plus they're inexpensive.

Spices: A well-stocked spice rack is one of the easiest ways to enhance your meal's flavor without adding fat or calories. Many spices contain unique health benefits from warding off the common cold to easing digestive discomfort. If you're just building your spice cabinet, start with the basics—salt, pepper, garlic powder, oregano, cinnamon, red pepper flakes, smoked paprika, cumin, chili powder, and curry powder.

The Refrigerator

Avocados: Rich in healthy fats, fiber, and antioxidants, avocados are a "superfood" you should have on hand to mash on toast, add to smoothies, turn into sauces and dressings, throw in a salad, or use in burgers like the Tuna Avocado Burgers. When shopping finds, avocados that are soft to squeeze, but not mushy. If you remove the stem at the top, it should be green, not brown.

Eggs: Eggs are a quick, easy, and versatile protein source to stock in your refrigerator. When possible, look for the terms "organic," "free-range," and "no added hormones." Although "pasture-raised" is not a regulated term, these eggs have been found to contain more anti-inflammatory omega-3 fatty acids and vitamin D.

Fresh fish and shellfish: You'll learn how to select the best fish later in the, but always ask your fishmonger what's freshest when at the fish counter.

Fresh herbs: Add fresh herbs for a bright burst of flavor and plenty of health benefits. Parsley, cilantro, dill, rosemary, and thyme are just a few favorites featured throughout the recipes in this book.

Fruit: Most Americans do not consume the recommended two to three servings of fruit per day. Stock your refrigerator with your favorites, so you always have an easy snack option. Berries, apples, and pears contain the most fiber but also shop for melons, bananas, and stone fruits for variety.

Organic tofu: Tofu is an excellent source of plant-based protein and calcium, which is why it's perfect for the pescatarian diet. Organic tofu is inexpensive and GMO-free.

Vegetables: You can't go wrong when stocking your refrigerator with vegetables. When shopping, your cart should look like a rainbow.

The Freezer

Frozen fish: Frozen fish is an affordable way to incorporate seafood into your diet. Minimal nutrients, if any, are lost in the freezing process.

Frozen fruit: Frozen fruit is typically more affordable than fresh, and it's an excellent option for off-season fruit. It's picked and frozen at its peak ripeness, which also means its peak nutrient content.

Frozen vegetables: If you often let fresh vegetables spoil, opt for frozen! Picked, processed, and frozen at their peak ripeness, frozen plants are an excellent alternative to raw.

The Hardware

You don't need a Michelin-star-worthy kitchen to follow the pescatarian diet. Aside from an oven and stove, plus necessary kitchen utensils (like a spatula, spoon, and tongs), here are five kitchen essentials that will help you eat the pescatarian way:

Nesting mixing bowls: Whether you're making a salad, mixing cookie dough, or prepping vegetables to roast, a set of nesting mixing bowls will be helpful in your kitchen. If possible, find a game with matching lids for secure storage in your refrigerator.

For easy cleanup, parchment paper is a must-have in your pescatarian kitchen. Line sheet pans with parchment paper when roasting vegetables or baking fish to reduce cleaning time. Preparing fish en papillote, or in a pouch made from parchment paper, is a quick and straightforward technique.

Sauté pan or cast-iron pan: The best way to get crispy skin on fish is to pan-sear it on your stovetop. A heavy sauté pan or cast-iron pan is the best kitchen tool to use for this. Bonus points if your container is oven safe!

Sharp chef's knife: Investing in a good chef's knife, and knowing how to use it, will make prep time a breeze! A good knife has a sturdy cutting board that doesn't slide with each cut.

Sheet pans: Whether you're roasting, baking, or broiling, sheet pans are necessary to get the job done. Look for rimmed sheet pans to prevent spills in your oven.

Smart Spending

The pescatarian diet can cost a pretty penny since seafood is one of the most expensive proteins available. You can be a smart shopper and spend less, however, by following these tips:

- Plan your meals to avoid waste. Making your own, you'll prevent food waste and buy only what you need and use for the week.

- Choose frozen over fresh. Frozen seafood, vegetables, fruit, and even grains can be more affordable than their new counterparts. Much of the fish you see "fresh" at the fish counter was frozen (check the signs and ask your fishmonger). Even more, you don't have to worry about waste as much when buying frozen foods, since they last longer and don't have to be used right away.

- Eat seasonally. In-season produce and fish are less expensive, so plan your meals accordingly. The crab season is in the fall and winter. Reserve your crab intake for these months to get the biggest bang for your buck!

- Use a bulk frozen fish delivery service. Several frozen food delivery services allow you to purchase high-quality fish and shellfish in bulk at discounted prices. Frozen is just as nutritious as fresh, so don't be shy about using these services (if you have the freezer space).

- Shop for staples online. Frequently, buying nonperishable staples, including dry grains, canned beans, canned tomatoes, canned fish, and oil online, can save you money. Just as you may price-compare your local supermarkets, shop around online between different vendors to find the best deals.

Selecting and Preparing Fish And Seafood

Is preparing fish and shellfish intimidating to you? You're not alone.

Maybe it's the scaly skin, hard shells, or googly eyes staring back at you. Perhaps it's fear of a fishy scent lingering throughout your home. Or maybe attempts resulted in a dry, overpriced home experiment that didn't turn out favorably. Whatever fishy beliefs you may have, purchasing, preparing, and cooking seafood are much easier than you think.

You don't have to worry about many of these common obstacles if you're just getting started. There are foolproof ways to master cooking fish at home.

First, choose a doable recipe. Instead of cooking a whole fish, try baking a flaky fish fillet, like the <u>Slow-Roasted Dijon Arctic Char</u>. In place of preparing mussels or clams, choose a more natural shellfish, like peeled and deveined shrimp, to boost your confidence. Get help at the fish counter. You don't need to fillet and debone your fish to be successful. Second, choose an affordable option to ease your fears of wasting money. Start with frozen or canned seafood to get your feet wet. Last, be sure to stay focused in the kitchen. Fish has a short cooking time, making it easy to go from flaky fillet to dry and overcooked quickly, but there's no need to be intimidated. Don't leave the kitchen while your fish cooks and avoid multitasking. As a guide, your fish is fully cooked when it becomes opaque and the flesh flakes when pressed with a fork.

And remember, if at first, you don't succeed, try and try again. There are so many fish varieties available; the fish counter is your oyster (pun intended)!

Chapter 6: Prepping for The Ketogenic Diet

At this point, you are surely eager to get started with the Keto diet. Whether you have chosen to follow the SKD or any of the other types, you will find that making the most of your chosen approach. That is why this is focused on helping you get the most out of your new eating plan by keeping in mind some fundamental guidelines and recommendations.

So, do take the time to go over this while considering the finer points of the Keto diet. You will surely find that making the most of your diet plan will help you achieve your goals in far less time than you might initially think it could take.

Importance of Nutrition on the Ketogenic Pescatarian Diet

The first part of success on the Ketogenic Pescatarian Diet is learning how to hone in on your nutrition. As we have throughout this book, the Ketogenic Pescatarian Diet is a low-carb, moderate-protein, high-fat diet. While there are many moving parts to this diet, it is essential that you master the basics before you try to get fancy with your results. Following the basic rules of the food, you will find you are going to start losing weight like you never thought was possible.

As a regular woman, losing weight might seem like an uphill battle. Later in this book, you will find delicious recipes to help fuel your health instead of harming it. Through nutrition alone, you will be able to improve your health but paired with a proper exercise program, and you will reach those results even quicker!

Remember that before you begin your diet, it is going to be vital that you find your macronutrients to help you reach your goals. If you are genuinely looking for life-changing results, these numbers cannot just be guessed.

Getting your body into ketosis takes a proper science. As you will recall from the first book, we all have a different carbohydrate limit. When you find your limit, you will discover how easy or hard it will be for you to get into ketosis.

Importance of Exercise on Ketogenic Pescatarian Diet

At this moment, you probably already realize that diet and exercise is essential for your health. While this is true, the combination of the two is going to be a bit more complicated than that while following the ketogenic diet. For this reason, you will have to be a bit more mindful about your new lifestyle, especially if you are just starting on the Ketogenic Diet.

When you begin restricting carbs in your diet, this is going to cause a chain-reaction of changes within your body. Some of these changes that occur may affect your performance when it comes to exercise; this is why it is going to be so crucial that you are cautious with your choices. You see, by restricting carbohydrates, you will be limiting your muscle cells from access to sugar as per usual. When your cells are lacking this sugar, your muscles will no longer be able to function at high intensities.

For this reason, athletes are typically on a less-strict version of the Ketogenic Diet. If you are looking to lose weight, the good news is that you will be able to do this with diet alone. By incorporating exercise, you will be able to maximize your results without needing crazy exercise routines.

The key to success here is going to be finding your perfect macronutrients to fuel your exercise routines. As you can see, these two elements of a healthier lifestyle are going to go hand in hand!

Before You Begin the Ketogenic Pescatarian Diet

Before you begin your diet, I invite you to take a few moments to think about your why. WHY are you looking to change your life? Are you improving your experience for yourself? Is it for your children? Your Grandchildren? We all have a different reason as to why we want to become healthier. I want you to use your why to fuel your success while following the Ketogenic Diet.

Remember that for anyone, weight loss is going to be a prolonged process. This is why it is so easy for people to give up before they reach their goal. Every time you think about giving up or cheating on your diet, think about your why and get right back on track.

Before you begin planning for your diet, try to set yourself up for success. The very first step is going to be setting realistic goals for yourself. If you give yourself an unattainable goal, you are already setting yourself up for failure. As you select your personal goals for your diet, focus on small benchmarks. An example of this would be to eat one good meal in a day or lose five pounds in the first month. When you hit your goals because they are attainable, this gives you a burst of confidence to keep going!

With that in mind, remember that there is no reason for you to change your lifestyle overnight! Up until this point, you have probably lived your life in a very particular way. While this may not be what is best for you, nobody is expecting you to blow up your metabolism and just be healthier all of a sudden! You will raise your chances of success by taking the race slow and steady. Even if you just start by lowering your calorie intake by 200 calories, you will still lose weight! By making it slow, you will avoid burning yourself out.

Speaking of burning yourself out, remember that there is no reason to be a perfectionist on your new diet. You are going to experience some setbacks! Remember that your body is going to go through some significant changes. When you think about it, it is pretty amazing you can run off of fat instead of glucose in the first place. As you go through the process, remember to be kind to yourself, and when you experience a setback, take a breath, and keep going!

For some, your motivation may be enough for you, but if not, it is always an excellent idea to find a buddy to experience this with! You may be surprised how many people out there have similar goals to yours. It is essential to have a support group while following the new diet to call on for motivation and a boost in your willpower. This way, when you hit one of those speedbumps or are suffering through the keto flu, you have someone to go through it with. When you are in something together, you will end up on the other side as more energetic individuals.

Finally, remember to be patient and reward yourself for all of the excellent work you are putting into yourself. When you think about it, the weight you have now didn't just happen overnight. Your weight loss is going to take a while, too, but the important part is that you are doing something about it!

The truth is, dieting is hard work for everyone, and sometimes, it just isn't any fun! A way to keep yourself going through the tough times is to give yourself a small reward! As you set your mini-goals for your weight loss, reward yourself with mini bonuses! Whether you reward yourself with a bubble bath, a new pair of pants, or a great massage, celebrate the small things!

At this point, I hope you are feeling motivated and excited to begin your new journey on the Ketogenic Diet. It is going to take work, and it is going to be hard at times, but you can get through anything! Once you get the basics down and get into a routine, the only thing you will be asking yourself is, why didn't you start sooner!

Remember that at the end of this book, you will be provided with meal plans and exercise routines. While they are just suggestions, they will stand as a great building block for you. Eventually, you will be able to write your plans based on your personal goals.

Set your goals in writing

When you write down your goals, you are making a written contract with yourself. This written contract will allow you to keep yourself accountable to… well, yourself. You don't need to be responsible for anyone else. You know who you are, what you want, and where you want to be. That is why it is of the utmost importance for you to become aware of what you need to accomplish.

With that in mind, some folks find it useful to keep a journal. It doesn't have to be much. It could even be an excel spreadsheet with dates and ideas. In this journal, you can keep track of what you are doing and your achievements. So, if you are looking to lose weight, you can track your influence. If you are looking to improve your stamina, you can keep track of your workouts. Or, if you are looking to improve health, you can keep track of the medication you are taking. You might be surprised to find that your doctor may even begin to cut back on your meds.

But all of this begins with your ability to stay on track. To do so, you need to have a clear picture of what your goals look like. After all, how far would you get if you hopped in your car and just drove? You might not get very now. But if you are clear on where you are going, even if it will take you days to reach your destination, you will eventually get there.

Reaching your ultimate goal is a matter of focus and dedication. This is not a sprint. This is more like a marathon. And as any marathon runner will tell you, you need to pace yourself. By walking yourself, you will eventually get to where you want to be. You might not be in the first place, but just the satisfaction of finishing the race might make it seem like you were the winner.

Chapter 7: Mistakes to Avoid on A Ketogenic Diet

I need to cover some of the mistakes that I frequently see humans make on a ketogenic food regimen. If you can keep away from those errors, you will be much more likely to shed pounds and feel better.

Mistake #1: Bad Mindset

Many human beings deal with the Ketogenic Pescatarian Diet as something they'll "attempt for a week or two."

They want to dip their toe within the water to look if the weight loss program "works." But they don't want to commit.

There are two problems with this technique. If you're no longer committed, then you are going to give up at the first signal of hassle. If you get tempted or do not lose weight for some days, you may give it all up. And I can assure you that now not the entirety will move flawlessly for you. It by no means does.

The second hassle is that no weight loss program works except your technique as a lifestyle.

If you need, you could lose a few weights after which pass again to ingesting bread, pasta, and sugar. But in case you move back to consuming the one's ingredients, you'll also give lower back to gaining weight. That is what we name the yo-yo dieting trap.

Mistake #2: Eating Too Much

Many people have developed bad eating habits. We'll consume until the whole thing is long past on our plates, we're going to devour when it is mealtime as opposed to when we're hungry. And we're going to snack all day instead of consuming actual meals.

All of this, unfortunately, leads to a variety of overeating.

Mistake #3: Not Testing

Our bodies are all a bit one-of-a-kind. Two human beings eating the equal Ketogenic Pescatarian Diet can now and again get specific results.

One man or woman could be in ketosis and dropping weight, and another character could be struggling.

That's why testing is so important. You want to ensure that you're without a doubt in ketosis. And if you aren't, then you could make modifications to your weight loss program and life.

When you're in ketosis, your frame will produce ketone our bodies. There are three varieties of ketone our bodies: Acetoacetate (AcAc), Beta-hydroxybutyrate (BHB), and Acetone.

In your blood, you may degree all three ketones our bodies. In your urine, AcAc and Acetone can be measured. And for your breath, simply Acetone.

Your blood ketone degrees are an excellent indicator of ketosis. Unfortunately, measuring blood ketone levels is also the most high-priced method.

That's why many humans still degree their urine and breath ketone ranges alternatively.

For weight loss, you don't need to chase high ketone ranges measuring and tracking ketones is just another way to get more records about what's occurring for your body, so do not get caught on ketone levels!

Mistake #4: Not Eating Enough Nutrient-Dense Foods

On a ketogenic weight loss plan, you'll pay several attentions to the macronutrients you devour, and you can use our Keto Calculator to figure out the right share of fats, carbs, and protein for you: keto summit keto-calculator

But consider that you also need to be getting enough nutrients and minerals.

You might be aware of some terrible matters that happen in case you're critically deficient in a micronutrient. For example,

You can get scurvy in case you don't get sufficient vitamin C.

You can get goiter if you're deficient in iodine.

Or you could cross blind in case you don't get sufficient diet A.

Another amazing test to take into account is a DEXA scan. This test will degree your fats ranges in addition to your bone and muscle degrees. If you do it before you begin your food plan, you will be able to music later, precisely how properly your food plan is working.

Besides those acute issues, continual deficiencies also can be a huge hassle. Often, nutrient deficiencies are not so severe which you exhibit a specific disease. That doesn't mean, though, that they may be not making you less healthy.

Over time, if you're low in nutrients and minerals, your frame just may not feature well. That can result in illnesses, fatigue, and more significant. Even minor nutrition and mineral deficiencies are probably making it more robust so one can shed pounds.

A smooth manner to enhance your micronutrient intake is to consume more nutrient-dense ingredients. Most of those foods in shape nicely right into a ketogenic eating regimen.

For instance, inexperienced leafy vegetables, organ meats, and seafood are all ketogenic-friendly. And they maybe some of the most nutrient-dense meals you could devour.

Supplementation with a terrific multivitamin or veggies powder is likewise helpful.

If you're into checking out, then attempt getting a SpectraCell evaluation, or a Urine Organic Acid take a look at. Both of these assessments will tell you which vitamins and minerals you are deficient in. That way, you can focus mainly on those deficiencies.

Mistake #5: Eating Toxic, Inflammatory Foods - Even if They're Low Carb

Not everything low in carbs is right for you. Period.

For example, you can go to maximum grocery stores these days and discover low-carb processed ingredients. You can get low-carb bread, low-carb cookies, and low-carb snacks.

You might be capable of stay in ketosis while consuming the one's low-carb foods, but they may be nonetheless awful for your body. Many of them contain wheat, gluten, and different inflammatory components.

And as I mentioned, the inflammation usually makes it more difficult for you to shed pounds.

Here are components that I recommend avoiding, even in low-carb meals:

Wheat, Rye, and Barley. The new era has created a manner to make these foods low-carb on occasion. But they nevertheless always include gluten, so one can inevitably motive irritation to your frame. Plus, they are not very nutrient-dense.

Dairy. Yes even cheese. In summary, dairy is probably ok. The hassle is which you do not live in an abstract world. Milk will pretty much always hold you out of ketosis. And the vast majority of humans have some degree of sensitivity to dairy products like cheese. (This is maximum probably actual even in case you are not lactose-intolerant.) Plus, you are in all likelihood to overeat cheese and cream!

Vegetable and Seed Oils. This includes Vegetable Oil, Canola Oil, Corn Oil, Sunflower Oil, and similar merchandise. Your cooking oil also makes a significant distinction in your weight loss. As Dr. Shanahan points out in her book, Deep Nutrition, those oils produce trans-fats, which can block your enzymes for burning fats.

Any food you have an intolerance to. Start paying greater interest to your body. If you wake up sooner or later and notice which you're congested or that your joints are stiff, ask yourself what you ate. You're possibly touchy to one of the meals you ate the day earlier than.

Also, be careful with nuts. Many people have allergies or sensitivities to nuts. But extra than that, nuts are easy to overeat. A ketogenic weight-reduction plan is not magic, so consuming 3,000 energy of nuts in step with day goes to make a difference.

Mistake #6: Ignoring Sleep, Exercise, and Stress

While ingesting a proper diet is essential for weight loss, it's not all that matters. Much weight-loss research has pressured the importance of sleep (7+ hours), exercise, and destressing. It's tough to get everything proper all at once. Still, any small efforts you make in those areas can pay off inside the end.

Mistake #7: Not Being Patient

So if you're going to give the ketogenic eating regimen a strive, then simply supply it a try to be patient.

It's taken you a lifetime of eating poorly to get to where you're at. You can't assume to repair all that harm in only a few weeks.

Mistake #8: Not Eating Enough Fiber

Mainstream vitamins have gotten a lot of things wrong.

The importance of fiber is not one of them. The past few years of scientific research have shown simply how crucial thread is for your intestine health.

In particular, soluble fiber and resistant starches from veggies can enhance your gut bacteria. Fermented ingredients like sauerkraut are additionally exquisite in this regard.

And in case you have problem-consuming enough veggies, then take a tremendous prebiotic like the CoBionic Foundation.

Chapter 8: Weight Loss and Exercise

We all know that exercise is right for you and that it can help you lose weight, but we don't necessarily do it. Many individuals are giving the excuse that they don't want to be huge and bulky or don't have enough time; the truth isn't many people like to exercise and get bored. You will learn a simple workout that you can do in no time; thus, you won't have any excuse to practice anymore. Exercise keeps you healthy, glad, and enables you to sleep much more accessible.

Contrary to the common faith, working out on days of fasting can effectively lead to a higher level of muscle building and fat burning than working out on average days. Noradrenaline concentrations are higher when fasting, enabling you to practice harder while increasing the attention of human growth hormones assist in boosting muscle mass. Misinformed and uninformed individuals indicate that fasting lowers muscle mass, which is not a fact.

If you want to burn fat by following any diet or regiment, one fact that remains constant is that you have to take fewer calories than you burn. You need to generate a calorie deficit of that quantity to lose a certain amount. You can't locate a fat-burning post or book and forget the term ' calories,' so what are they? These are food's energy. Calories power every action in your body, so your body needs them always.

Calories are obtained from carbohydrates, fats, and proteins and are your body's primary source of energy. They are either used as physical energy or deposited as body fat regardless of where they came from. Stored calories will remain as fat in your body unless used up by reducing the intake of calories so that your body can use up the reserves or burn more calories than you take in by physical exercise. It's excellent for you to exercise and make you feel good.

How do you calculate the calories you eat, the calories you need to burn, and the calories you burned during your workout? Check the nutritional content of the food supplied on the back or side of the box to calculate the calories in the food you bought from the store. There are distinct quantities of calories per unit in each macronutrient. Twenty grams of protein include four calories, 35 grams of carbohydrate contains four calories, and 15 grams of fat add nine calories. Calculate the food's calorific value by multiplying the caloric equal of each macronutrient. These nutrients are always calculated in grams. To discover the complete calories of the meals, add the calories provided off by each macronutrient. When calculating the number of calories like this, you will not only find out the calorific value but also incorporate it into a balanced diet. The serving size and the number of servings contained must be taken into account. Nearly all of them indicate only one serving's calorific amount, the number of meals can alter the calorie count. Always compare the number of nutrients you are taking with the recommended values, so you don't eat too much or too little. Online calculators and guide books can also be used to help you do this.

You should first know your basal metabolic rate to know how many calories you burn during the workout session. This is the amount of energy that your body uses to work. There is no constant number because everything depends on several factors. Age is one of the determining factors for your BMR. The older you are, the lower your BMR, the more exercise you will need. A muscular person is more likely to burn more fat than a fat person. The ambient temperature also serves apart as the higher your BMR will be. The hotter it is, the higher your BMR is this because you are warmed up by the setting, so more calories are invested in losing weight. Work out duration is also a significant factor, the better, the longer, but don't overdo it. The fitter you are, the fewer calories you will consume as your body is already used to it. Your diet has a direct effect on your metabolism. If you don't consume enough, drink too much, or exercise any other poor dietary habits, your metabolism will be impacted, thus decreasing the number of calories you burn. Lack of sufficient sleep can cause you to consume more calories as you become more exhausted, and practice is more probable, but it can also impact your metabolism. Oxygen helps to offer energy to your body to continue to work. You will consume more calories if you breathe more strongly during workouts.

Some conventional methods are available to approximate the number of calories you burn in a day. Everyone has their strengths and weaknesses, so it's best to use them all and use the mean as the estimate for the best results. The first is by using exercise devices such as the Fit bit to monitor your regular motions and assess calories consumed during the period they are held. While it has been discovered that the number of calories burned is not entirely precise, they are convenient and straightforward. Metabolic screening is another technique. The machinery needed for this technique in laboratories and clinics can be accessed affordably from there as they are costly. These examinations can assist you in changing what you eat and your exercise regiment, but some individuals do not think the price of this technique is worth it. Always try to ensure that a skilled technician tests you so you can get the most accurate results. The last but mostly used is online calculators. These calculators are trying to offer your weekly spending an estimated value. The amount they offer is very general, but they can be used as your weight loss guideline. Calculating the mean of all these techniques will provide you with a near assessment of how many calories you consume in a day.

Yes, exercising on an empty stomach is okay and secure. A generally healthy adult can usually practice on an empty stomach without having any adverse reactions. Working out without eating will result in you burning more body fat. You are more likely to have more energy when you're in a fasted state to do your workout routine.

However, if you have experienced fainting, feeling dizzy, or weak after practice during a fasted state, do not continue doing it. Always listen to your body; without even knowing it, you might destroy it. By organizing an exercise timetable that operates well with your fasting timetable as you can organize your time table in any direction you like, you can manage around this. Fasted exercise can speed up the weight loss process.

There is a fat-burning myth that you have to eat fat to lose body fat when you exercise. At first, it may seem embarrassing why discovering reality is not real but read on. People believe that when carrying out an aerobic workout that encourages peak fat loss, there is a particular sweet spot. During low-intensity practice, a higher quantity of fat is used, but the entire amount of fat used is low. Increasing exercise intensity improves the amount of fat used.

The impacts of various intensities of aerobic exercise have been likened, and the typical finding is that the total fat loss is equivalent regardless of the strength at which the practice was performed, provided the caloric consumption is the same. This implies that the quantity of calories used during training is more essential than the energy used. The body decreases fat as soon as it burns more calories than it eats. Exercise intensity and length are inversely proportional. The higher the concentration of activity requires, the lower the workout length. For a lengthy period of high-intensity exercise for a brief period, you can attempt a low-intensity task to fit your body best.

If you want a healthy heart and lungs, you should look after your body. Strength training is essential. There's no doubt that organizations make you feel beautiful, and they also help you burn calories while you're sleeping. If you enhance your muscle amount, your sensitivity to insulin will also increase. To help boost your muscle mass, you should develop a fitness exercise scheme to reduce your weight and improve muscle mass.

During aerobic exercise, the calorie expenditure is average, five calories/minute during a low-intensity workout, and around ten calories/minute during a high-intensity workout. Two exercise days, even if you burn more calories, do not equal the fat-burning of losing calories across several days. You should exercise like three times/week, but the division between weights, interval training, and weights depends on your goals.

If you do exercise, but you do not change your diet, your weight loss process will be prolonged. It is not easy to reach a point that the amount of fat you will burn will be directly proportional to the amount and time you spend exercising. About nine calories/minute are used during weight training. On top of burning calories through exercise, there are also more calories lost after the practice, which is called excess post-exercise oxygen consumption. It is due to an increase in adrenalin and noradrenalin on top of other factors that make your system burn calories even after exercise from the fat stores. The magnitude of the post-exercise calorie loss is dependent on the intensity and duration in which the activity was carried out. Not many people can be able to sustain energy to the point that they generate a large EPOC.

Dieting without exercise is a common approach people undertake. The problem with it is that it leads to a loss in lean body mass and reduced metabolic rate. To make up for the calorie restriction, the system lowers the metabolic rate. As a result, your body can enter starvation mode; thus, you will not lose weight. When food intake is returned, the lowered metabolism results in regain of the fat that was lost. It is not an effective long term plan. If you eat too little and exercise more, you may enter into starvation mode, which can stop fat loss completely. Achieving the equilibrium between exercise and dietary alterations to enhance weight loss while preventing muscle loss is the ultimate goal. Getting more muscular will raise your metabolic rate.

High-interval intensity training, HIIT, is an exercise method that works incredibly with to promote weight loss and results in more significant weight loss than lower intensity continuous workout. You simply switch between periods of high-intensity activity and periods of low-intensity exercise. The practice can suit your timetable, however tight your schedule is. It allows you in a short time to get the advantages of lengthy workout sessions. There are different kinds of intermittent fasting you can attempt. If you like cycling, you could: warm-up with soft cycling, start pedaling after a minute as you do and boost the strength, after 15 seconds your bodies get tired, if you can proceed at the same speed then the power you set is not big enough, you will discover your ideal fierce resistance after practicing severely after fast-cycling reduces the strength. By walking, swimming, and any other workout that can be performed quickly, you can also do HIIT without a bicycle.

Chapter 9: Strict Diet for Fat Burning

Eat More Cruciferous Vegetables

Incorporate more cruciferous veggies like broccoli and cauliflower in your diet. This group of vegetables is known as the crucifers, in light of the flowers that often sprout looking like a cross. They contain an assortment of healthy mixes, including sulforaphane, founded by Dr. Paul Talley, M.D., at Johns Hopkins University. Talley distinguished this specific compound in broccoli, taxi bagel, watercress, and other cruciferous vegetables as having the best ability to deliver detoxifying proteins. He later found that broccoli sprouts, which appear as though horse feed sprouts, however, are not as thready, have ten to one hundred times more sulforaphane than broccoli does.

Cruciferous vegetables incorporate the following:

Arugula Bok choy Broccoli Broccolini

Broccoli rabe Broccoli sprouts

Brussels sprouts Cabbage Cauliflower Chinese cabbage Collard greens Kale

Mustard greens Rutabaga

Swiss chard Turnip greens Turnips Watercress

Sulforaphane, a cell reinforcement, accelerates the detoxification of numerous conceivably unsafe synthetic compounds, upgrades glutathione production, and is accepted to forestall malignant growth and stifle tumor development.

Another compound in crucifers called indole carbinol has been found to build the detoxification of estrogen in the liver by as much as 50 percent. This makes it incredibly gainful during weight loss when the liver is immersed with estrogen-like synthetics from fat stores. Indole carbinol is also accepted to battle disease, particularly bosom and prostate malignant growth.

How to Do It: Aim for in any event two servings of cruciferous vegetables per day (1 serving = 1/2 cup cooked, 1 cup crude, or 1/4 cup broccoli sprouts). One route is to add arugula to your serving of mixed greens. While the more significant part of us consider arugula an option in contrast to lettuce, it's a cruciferous vegetable. It contains more vitamin C and calcium than some other plate of mixed greens green, along with folic acid and other vitamins and minerals. On the off chance that you locate arugula's impactful, peppery bite to be a bit overpowering, search for child arugula, which is less spicy and hot, or have a go at blending it in with other serving of mixed greens to soften the taste. Arugula servings of mixed greens taste good with dressings made with lemon juice, balsamic vinegar, extra virgin olive oil, or hazelnut oil.

Another option is cauliflower, one of the couples of cruciferous vegetables (along with turnips) that can be utilized as a substitute for boring foods. Take a stab at hacking it finely in the food processor to reenactor the surface of the rice, or squashing it—a more beneficial option as it contains about 33% of the calories of potatoes. Attempt the flavorful Chicken Stir-fry over the "Rice" formula in this book, which utilizes cauliflower rather than rice. My favorite method to eat cauliflower is as a snack. I slash it into bitesize pieces, hurl it with extra virgin olive oil and a bit of ocean salt, and meal it in the grill until it's gently caramelized. You can include cumin, cayenne, or other flavors since enormous quantities can debilitate thyroid function. Any cooking, whether it's steaming, bubbling, heating, broiling, barbecuing, or microwaving, deactivates the undesirable thyroid impeding mixes.

Eat-in Color

The shade of each fruit and vegetable offers more than aesthetic intrigue. We can categorize a plant's specific nutritional worth dependent on its color, which is brought about by phytonutrients or plant supplements.

Each color sneaks up suddenly as far as your body's ability to get more fit.

The Purple Protectors (Purple or Red)

This gathering contains anthocyanins (pronounced a homomer union), water-soluble cell reinforcements that diminish the danger of malignant growth, coronary illness, diabetes, and hypersensitivities, and forestall DNA harm, inflammation, and untimely maturing. A vital piece of the diet, this gathering has the following explicit benefits:

Has characteristic calming properties that improve insulin and leptin sensitivity

Strengthens veins and vessels, decreasing varicose veins and cellulite formation

Helps forestall obesity

Is high in fiber (particularly raspberries)

Reduces the breakdown of collagen by inflammatory synthetic concoctions, which anticipates skin maturing

Beets Blackberries Black Currants Blueberries Cherries

Cranberries Eggplant Plums Pomegranates Purple cabbage

Raspberries Red apple Strawberries

Beets are stacked with betaine, a liver securing cancer prevention agent that has been found to help the liver procedure fats and keep fat from accumulating in the liver. In one investigation, betaine supplements fundamentally improved liver catalysts and diminished fat deposits in the liver. Creature concentrates also show that betaine can improve liver function and secure against chemical harm to the liver.

Blueberries are one of the highest in cell reinforcements of any fruit or vegetable. They contain the phytochemical anthocyanidins and are wealthy in gelatin, the fiber that ties to poisons and also helps lower cholesterol. Blueberries also have a compound like cranberries, called epic ate jawline, and can be utilized to forestall urinary tract infections.

Raspberries, strawberries, and pomegranates contain ellagic corrosive and intensify that has been found to secure against liver harm, improve glutathione, kill poisons, and diminish the weight impacts of endocrine disruptors.

Raspberries are especially useful for you. As of late, Japanese scientists isolated a compound in raspberries that has one of a kind weightless impact. They gave creatures a high-fat diet for ten weeks. They found that supplementing the menu with the raspberry compound diminished stomach fat, triglycerides, all-out muscle to fat ratio, and by and substantial weight, and improved their ability to consume fat.

How to Do It:

Each day, eat at any rate one serving (1 serving = 3⁄4 cup) of the purple protectors, whether it includes a handful of new or solidified berries to your morning meal, getting a charge out of straightforward, however delightful sweet!

Have a go at having beets with supper. Beets can be bubbled, pureed, roasted, flame-broiled, or cured. Bubble them unpeeled and leave an inch of the green stem in any event, so the color doesn't drain. Raw beets can be ground into plates of mixed greens or squeezed with other vegetables. Opportunity to cook them, search for canned beets at the market. Keep away from jostled beets, which as a rule, accompany included sugar. Beets have a hearty sweetness that is best supplemented in plates of mixed greens by vinaigrette with lemon, apple juice vinegar, or balsamic vinegar, and intense flavors, for example, arugula, olives, and feta cheddar.

If you are in a hurry, attempt unsweetened pomegranate juice, which has a dark red color and a tart taste, Blueberry juice is another option. You can drink the milk, or have a go at blending 1⁄4 cup of pomegranate squeezes in with a solitary serving of nonfat organic vanilla yogurt in a bowl for a snappy smoothie. Even though you lose the fiber by drinking rather than eating these fruits, you'll despite everything appreciate the other medical advantages of eating these purple protectors.

The Extraordinary Oranges (Yellow, Orange, or Green)

This is the biggest gathering, containing fat-soluble phytonutrients called carotenoids (pronounced vehicle rotenoids). As the name infers, these plant shades give carrots their orange color. This gathering includes vegetables and fruits running from yellow to green to orange because the green pigmented chlorophyll that provides plants with their trademark green color can dominate the orange shade in specific foods.

Beta-carotene is the most popular carotenoid. However, this gathering also incorporates other carotenoids, for example, lutein (pronounced Lehigh schooler), lycopene, alpha-carotene, and foods plentiful in vitamin C and the related bioflavonoids. The following vegetables and fruits contain carotenoids:

Vegetables Fruit

Ringer peppers Carrots Green beans Leafy greens Lettuce Peas, green Peppers Pumpkin Spinach Squash Sweet Potatoes Tomatoes Zucchini Apricots Cantaloupes

Clementine's Grapefruit, pink Guava Honeydew Kiwi Lemons Nectarines Oranges Passionfruit Peaches Pears Persimmons Tangerines Watermelon The amazing oranges do an assortment of essential functions required for weight loss.

They ensure our phone films (which are made out of more than 30 percent fat) and other tissues from poison harm during weight loss.

They improve the sensitivity of insulin.

In specific, lycopene, a carotenoid found in tomatoes, decreases the danger of cardiovascular infection.

The orange gathering also contains foods high in vitamin C, which is essential during weight loss for the following reasons:

Aids in the formation of the appetite suppress neurotransmitters serotonin and dopamine

Helps forestall pressure-related weight gain in the guts

Boosts glutathione levels and is associated with deactivating poisons

Reduces inflammation by affecting histamine discharge and degradation

It lowers the measure of cholesterol in bile by converting cholesterol to bile acids, making bile more averse to bunch together and forming stones.

Watermelon, red chime peppers, melon, and kiwi. Be that as it may, my top pick for vitamin C is guava. However, harder to discover in the supermarket than other fruits, guava, a yellowish-green tropical fruit, rates high in vitamin C. Search for guava in Asian markets and some supermarkets. Maintain a strategic distance from guava juice, which is sweetened.

How to Do It: Include in any event two servings (1/2 cup every one) of the fantastic oranges consistently. Have a go at including diced ringer peppers or solidified slashed spinach to a morning meal omelet, pressing grape or cherry tomatoes to have with lunch, or microwaving solidified peas, green beans, or a little sweet potato to have with your supper rather than a white potato. If you, as a rule, have a plate of mixed greens, have a go at grinding raw carrots into the serving of mixed greens and substituting spinach rather than lettuce.

Numerous individuals who appreciate cooking with garlic and onions, remembering more of these foods for your diet ought to be simple. The dynamic phytonutrient in this family, called allicin, has been shown to lower cholesterol and pulse, forestall malignant growth, and improve general wellbeing. Here are only a couple of the weightless and medical advantages of this flavorful gathering:

Lowers absolute cholesterol, increments healthy HDL cholesterol, and forestalls the unsafe oxidation of LDL cholesterol

Improves detoxification by expanding the production of glutathione, allowing for the powerful elimination of poisons and carcinogenic substances

Foods in this gathering are:

Chives Endives

Garlic Leeks

Onions Scallions

Shallots

How to Do It: Aim for at any rate one serving of the correct whites every day (1 serving = 1/4 cup or one clove of garlic). Onions, garlic, shallots, chives, and scallions upgrade the flavor of various foods. If the idea of eating raw garlic causes you to wince, start with one clove, which despite everything, gives you a good measure of allicin (in any event 10 mg); however, generally doesn't bring about a perceivable garlic door. It should be squashed or hacked and added to food to discharge the allicin, rather than eaten entirety.

Chapter 10: Reaching Your Goal

The saying remains true — you will realize that what you put into your body is going to dictate how you feel. While on the Keto diet, you are building up energy stores for your body to utilize. This means that you should be feeling a necessary boost in your energy levels and the ability to get through each moment of each day without struggling. You can say goodbye to the sluggish feeling that often accompanies other diet plans. When you are on Keto, you should only be experiencing additional energy and unlimited potential. Your diet isn't going to always feel like a diet. After some time, you will realize that you enjoy eating a Keto menu very much. Because your body will be switching the way it metabolizes, it will also be switching what it craves. Don't be surprised if you end up craving fats and proteins as you progress on the Keto diet — this is what your body will eventually want.

Tracking Progress

Using a compare and contrast method is always great for tracking progress. Remember how you felt before starting the Keto diet. If you haven't started already, you can use this time to document your current state of being. Make sure to record your mindset and the cravings that you have. You can also mark down your current weight and BMI. When you have these figures to compare your progress to, you will be able to use this as a motivating tool. Remember to allow yourself to feel proud as you make it through each day of being on the Keto diet. Commit yourself and food. This will present its own set of challenges to face, but it is not going to be so complicated that you lose your way. Believe in your ability to see this through.

You Are What You Eat

Think about how you used to feel while eating your sugary and carb-loaded cravings. Your immediate response is likely going to suggest that you felt great but think about the bigger picture. Did you gain more energy from eating these things? Did you experience a crash after you ate them? Instant gratification might feel great at first, but you will likely have to deal with the consequences. Eating junk food only serves your immediate cravings. It also gets your body used to desire these things by reinforcing the behavior. Junk food holds no nutritional value, and it won't make you burn calories or use the sugar as a valid energy supply. When you think about it, this junk food indeed doesn't have a place in your life.

Know that you can obtain happiness in other ways that don't involve eating food. While eating does tend to be a social delight, it isn't the only thing that can make you happy when it comes to food. Choose to feel satisfied when you can know for sure that you are treating your body correctly. You should be able to handle the joy that comes from the fact that you are giving your body fuel that it can utilize. While eating your Keto-friendly food might not give you the same immediate rush eating your favorite junk food, it will benefit you much more in the long run. You will be able to notice its benefits long after you digest the food, and that is what is essential. A simple change in perspective is what you need to realize that your happiness isn't directly tied to the cravings that you satisfy. Your satisfaction needs to stem from a deeper place.

Eating tends to be an act of comfort when you are feeling down or worried. This is a cultural norm that many people experience. While being on the Keto diet, you will learn how to manage your emotions in a way that is not directly tied to the food you are eating. Instead of giving in to your cravings when you are having a hard day, the Keto diet teaches you to nourish yourself. When you are adequately fed, you will be able to boost your energy levels and maintain your endorphins.

As you know, this will be enough to give you some extra happiness when you need it. It is a more permanent solution to your problems that tend to linger. When you can think about things from this perspective, it will be easier to remember why you are on the Keto diet.

No diet should make you feel so miserable that you can't even enjoy its benefits. Keto is not a diet that should make you feel like you have no options. While on Keto, you should have the exact opposite experience. Because what you have to get rid of is minimal, you should be equipped with many different meals that you can enjoy on a guilt-free level. Diets that torment you emotionally are not suitable for you, no matter how healthy you are eating. With a healthy mind is just as important as having a healthy body. When your mindset begins to deteriorate, this will lessen your overall happiness levels. You are allowed to be happy while being on a diet! If you start to feel down, then something isn't right.

Through your example, other people will begin to see that Keto isn't as strict or complicated as they once thought. Being able to provide others with a real perspective can do a lot to keep the diet realistic. You can serve as an inspiration to your friends and loved ones to stick with your diet and remain happy and fulfilled. You may have likely tried to fake this feeling while being on nutrition in the past, but Keto does not involve any pretending. It is essential to listen to exactly how you are feeling and identify what makes you think this way. If you begin to experience anything negative, you are encouraged to alter your diet until you start to feel better. There should be no suffering while on the Keto diet!

Your Life Will Improve

There comes the point while being on the Keto diet that you make a shift from trying to succeeding. This will happen at various locations for people, but when it happens to you, embrace it. Instead of focusing on the fact that you are following a diet, you can begin to focus on the benefits you are receiving. You need to make sure that you are enjoying your life! There are so many things in life that try to get you down, so when you find something that brings you up, you should focus your attention on these things. One of the very first things that the Keto diet will provide you with is energy. As you have read, this is one of the benefits that you should experience reasonably quickly. Use your power to the best of your ability. Try to divide your time wisely, keeping in mind that the diet has allowed you some additional fuel to use throughout your day.

Even if you feel that your energy levels are currently on the rise, try to still practice healthy habits like going to bed earlier and waking up earlier. This is going to regulate your bodily systems further. What you need to remember is that the Keto diet is going to give you momentum. It is up to you to keep up with it. If you do nothing with it, then it is almost like these benefits are being wasted. When you can remain aware of them, you should be able to take full advantage of them. Try to practice as many healthy habits as you can when you first start noticing these new changes. This can be an exciting and uplifting time for you!

Chapter 11: Advantages and Disadvantages of Ketogenic Diet

Advantages of Keto Diet

The keto diet may have several positive effects on the body. One of the most prominent positive aspects of the keto diet is the ease of sticking to the food. Successful weight loss plans must be easy to follow for most people to be successful. A low-carb diet may be easy to follow because the keto diet can significantly reduce appetite. If you don't feel hungry, you're more likely to stay on the diet plan. When a person consumes carbohydrates, there is a burst of energy and a feeling of fullness. Unfortunately, these sensations are short-lived because the glucose used to generate energy burns away quickly. This leads to hunger within a short period. While on keto, the fats will keep you feeling full for a more extended period. Additionally, as long as you are snacking on items within the plan, there is much room for high-fat items in the diet.

Another good thing about the keto diet, especially in the beginning, you will lose weight. By staying on the plan and following the tenets, you're likely to lose up to twice as much weight at the beginning of a diet as you will with low-fat, low-calorie foods. This is especially true during the first two or three weeks on the menu as the body sheds excess water.

The keto diet reduces the amount of fat stored in the body. The fat loss is made up of visceral fat. Visceral fat is fat that accumulates in the abdomen and tends to attach itself to organs. The keto diet may reduce fat, which is known to be the most harmful and may reduce the risk of heart disease and type 2 diabetes. These issues are often seen in people who are obese or only overweight. The visceral fat loss reduces the fat in the most dangerous areas of the body and improves overall health in many individuals.

Ketogenic diets allow you to shed off extra weight without risking diseases rapidly. The Ketogenic Pescatarian Diet restricts the intake of carbohydrates, which forces your body into ketosis and, thus, a reduction of body fats. This diet helps you lose fat and ensures the mass of the muscles is well preserved. Ketogenic diets promote weight loss through an increase in intake of protein, which has numerous weight-loss advantages. The diet regulates carbohydrates' consumption, which is a crucial component in weight loss and burning calories as a result of the conversion of proteins and fats into ketone bodies that run your organization. The diet also assists in burning fats rapidly while taking part in physical exercises, during rests, and other ordinary days to day activities.

Control of Glucose in the Body

Another advantage of adopting the diet is that it can lower and regulate your blood sugar levels. Carbohydrates are responsible for the rise of blood sugar levels in your blood, and thus that threat is eliminated once you start on the Ketogenic diet. The Ketogenic Pescatarian Diet is known for its ability to reduceHbA1c – a known measure of your blood glucose control. This measure is significantly reduced by the diet of people who have type 2 diabetes.

The diet is also useful to the other types of diabetes, such as type 1 diabetes or LADA, and thus the diet should also regulate the glucose in your blood. It is important to note that if the food is maintained, the chances of controlling your blood's glucose could help reduce the risk of any other health complications from occurring.

A Reduction in Reliance on the Medication-Related to Diabetes

As you have already been aware of the diet's ability to reduce blood sugar levels, the menu also offers a chance to patients who have type 2 diabetes to reduce their reliance on medication. After a good while of sticking to it, the list will pay your efforts as you will be able to do away with the drug-related to type 2 diabetes, a study found. You could ultimately come off your medicine, or the diet could help reduce your dosage. However, consult with your doctor first before doing away with the mediation.

Control of High Blood Pressure

Numerous people in the world today are living and surviving with high blood pressure. With high blood pressure, your body becomes prone to several ailments, such as heart-related diseases, kidney-related diseases, or even stroke. The Ketogenic Pescatarian Diet helps you reduce the risk of all these diseases because the diet decreases your body's blood pressure levels if you are overweight or suffering from type 2 diabetes.

An improved Mental Performance

The diet will significantly improve your ability to remember and recall and improve your ability to focus. Ingestion of foods such as salmon, which are Keto-friendly, could boost your mood and your learning abilities in the classroom setting. The diet could also help enhance your long-term memory.

Restoration of Insulin Sensitivity

The Ketogenic Pescatarian Diet is known for removing the cause of insulin resistance as a consequence of elevated insulin levels in your body. The diet cuts on the ingestion of carbohydrates, leading to high levels of insulin in the body. With a reduction of insulin level in your body, the chances of burning fat in your body increases. This is because elevated levels of insulin interfere with the breaking down of fats.

Improved Cholesterol Levels

The Ketogenic Pescatarian Diet is a great agent in ensuring that your cholesterol levels in your blood are regulated. However, it is recommended to let your doctor of physician put you on the Keto diet if you intend to regulate your body's cholesterol levels. This is because this topic on cholesterol is complicated and would require qualified personnel to handle.

Satiety

The diet is also known for its ability to have a positive effect on your appetite. The moment your body succeeds in getting into ketosis, it becomes more comfortable with burning fats, which could, in turn, force your body to stop craving for food and thus improving your chances of doing away with overeating. In the long end, you would most likely succeed in losing weight.

Benefits to Individuals with Diabetes

Diabetes is a result of raised blood sugar levels, which, over time, are harmful to the heart, kidneys, nerves, and blood vessels. Diabetes manifests when the body is not in a position to produce adequate insulin, and if your body becomes tough to insulin. The diet comes in and eliminates this possibility. Ketogenic diets are essential in curbing type 2 diabetes, the most experienced type of diabetes among adults because the diet helps you shed extra fat, which is associated with this site type of diabetes. As a result of adapting to the menu for long periods, you could get off your medication.

Disadvantages of Keto Diet

Along with the dramatic change in diet, there may be some negative experiences on the ketogenic diet. One of the more common issues is keto flu. This is a general feeling of fatigue that may accompany entering ketosis. This feeling of tiredness may be accompanied by nausea and upset stomach. It is a common reaction to the body as it adapts to reduced carbohydrates and the switch to getting energy from ketones instead of glucose.

Besides the keto flu, there may also be keto diarrhea. This is likely caused by the gallbladder producing more bile to deal with increased fat consumption. Until the body adjusts to the increased amounts of fat and enters ketosis, diarrhea may be a side effect. Diarrhea may also result from a reduction in the number of fiber ingested because of a decrease in carbohydrate consumption. The tissue from carbs must be replaced with tissue from low-carb vegetables. This will help mitigate diarrhea issues resulting from the lack of carbohydrates and, therefore, the fiber in the diet.

One way to reduce gastrointestinal issues associated with the keto diet is to make sure you drink plenty of water. It is essential to stay hydrated and flush out your system. Drinking lots of water helps to remove toxins from the body before they have time to linger in organs and tissues.

The keto diet will precipitate weight loss. Unfortunately, this weight loss may include the reduction of muscle mass as well as fat. This is not ideal, especially for women over 50 in whom muscle mass begins to atrophy naturally. Additionally, reduced muscle mass may change your metabolism because you burn more calories with muscle than fat. This loss of tissue is more likely to happen if you are consuming more fat than protein. The type of fat consumed will be essential to retain muscle mass as you lose weight.

Chapter 12: The Best Ways to Lose Weight Fast

There are many ways you can approach losing weight. What is required is consistency and commitment. If you have been on a diet before, you will know that it will take a while to see results. This time to see your results will only lengthen as you age. Losing weight is not a race. It is a marathon.

Eat Out Less

Kirsten David, a dietitian with Edu Plated, explained that we are more prone to weight gain as we grow old. As mentioned in the, our metabolism slows down, and we undergo hormone change.

This sounds like a no-brainer, but you may be eating out more than you think. Other than the fact that you may be unwittingly digesting the food that dials your blood sugar to eleven, eating out is common among older adults, starting from age 50.

Due to mental, physical, or social barriers, you may be prevented from losing weight effectively. Many people at this age are either too mentally or physically tired to cook at home themselves. Plus, there are no more children in the house as they would be living on their elsewhere.

Without having any mouths to feed other than your own, going out and eating seems quite practical, right? Don't have to worry about thinking of what you should prepare for dinner, or having to stress about doing the dishes. But in reality, letting others control what you put into your mouth is one of the first mistakes in dieting. You put yourself at risk of consuming a higher amount of processed foods and high-fat foods.

Even for people in their 20's, eating the wrong food will get them fat quickly. At your age, the consequence of weight gain will increase drastically.

Instead, plan your meal. We will discuss how you can do that and which dishes to incorporate into your diet to help you lose weight, what to avoid.

Don't Skip Meals

On the flip side, skipping meals also leads to weight gain. Diet oversimplified would be "Eat less, move more," but you will not get the full effect. The statement is not accurate because you need to know exactly what food you need to cut down and what activity to partake.

In this case, let us talk about skipping meals. This leads to a drop in metabolism because when your body senses that you are not getting any food, it goes into power-saving mode.

As we age, our hormones change as well. Estrogen and testosterone, in particular, are affected, and this causes your body to process sugar efficiently. However, if you skip meals, your body will lack the critical nutrients needed, such as calories and protein.

Providing your body with enough calories or protein will maintain your muscle mass and regulate your hormones. Without them, your internal system will go haywire, and it won't be easy to steer everything back on track.

If it is inconvenient, then you do not have to eat three meals a day. So long as you get enough calories and nutrients every day, you should be fine. Avoid snacking because you won't be losing any weight when you graze on food all day long. Other than that, make sure to stay hydrated with fluids such as tea, water, or coffee.

Eat Less at Night

Some people have the habit of having dinner right before bedtime. Not only does that interfere with your body's digestion process, but you will also get the lower quality sleep that you need at your age. Many studies have shown that consuming fewer calories at night could help you maintain a slimmer, fitter body and shed excess fat.

You also put yourself at risk of developing metabolic syndrome, which can lead to heart disease, diabetes, and stroke because of your high blood sugar level and excess body fat.

So, keep most of the calories for breakfast and lunch. Keep dinner light to help you sleep tight.

Sleep

As mentioned before, sleep plays a huge role in hormone regulation, among other weight-related bodily functions. The key to getting enough sleep is establishing an asleep and morning routine. Do not look at blue lights (fluorescent, phone, computer) for at least 30 minutes before you go to sleep. If you must, you can download some applications for your device to make it produce orange light instead of blue. Orange lights are easier on your eyes and do not disrupt sleep.

Team Up

Getting into a new eating pattern or daily routine can be a challenge. Staying motivated requires even more willpower. Therefore, getting your friend, co-worker, or a family member to take up this new routine might give you a better chance to stick to your plan and achieve your goals.

Try Intermittent Fasting

Intermittent fasting is well-known because it does not change what you eat, but when and how often you do. Ditch the juice cleanses. The most common form is called the 16/8, but you do not have to do that. Instead, try fasting-mimicking. This form of fasting has been proven to improve your health. People who have tried this diet plan reported that they have lost six pounds on average, shredded up to two inches off their waistline, and significantly lowered their cancer risk.

Fasting-mimicking works because the nerves in your hypothalamus are damaged as you gain weight. They are responsible for conducting signals from your fat cells to your brain. When they are damaged, your mind does not know when you have eaten your fill. Therefore, you are prone to overeating.

However, when you give yourself some time away from eating, you let your hypothalamic nerves to rest and recuperate. That is why fasting-mimicking requires you to allocate five days out of every month to eat just between 750 to 1,000 calories, well below the recommended daily calorie intake. It sounds terrible to starve yourself, but you need to give your nerves a break to reset themselves.

Start friendly and manageable by eating only 800 calories twice a week, and your calorie sources for those days are primarily from vegetables, protein, and healthy oils (olive oils).

Of course, your stomach will feel empty on those days. To help alleviate this problem, consider following a low-carb diet as you fast. Thirty percent of your calories should come from protein, non-starchy veggies, beans, and nuts.

The best time to eat starchy carbohydrates is at the very end of the meal after your fill of veggies and protein. Doing this helps lower your blood sugar level and insulin as well as an increase of hormones to help you feel full for longer.

Please, download Intermittent Fasting After 50, if you are interested.

Mindful Eating

Sometimes, you do not even need to make that many changes. All you need is to put your attention in the right place as you eat. Your weight gain may be caused by stress. If that is the case, then you may need to practice mindful eating.

You might be overeating just because you are stressed. Therefore, practicing mindfulness techniques can be very helpful to help alleviate your anxiety and make you aware of how much you are eating.

Those who have practiced this technique are more successful in their weight loss efforts. Mindful eating requires you to pay attention to how full or hungry you feel, meal planning, focusing solely on your food tastes, and not doing anything else when you eat (such as watching TV).

To get started, just eat slowly. Place your fork between bites and take your time chewing your food. Focus on how it tastes and do not watch TV, look at your phone, or do anything other than eating.

The trick behind mindful eating is that your body takes time to detect when it is full. If you eat quickly, you already overate by the time your body realizes it is complete. Plus, it would be best if you took the time to enjoy tasty meals that you cook for yourself and reinforce the belief that your healthy home-cooked food helps your body maintain its youth.

Chapter 13: Weight Loss Affirmations

An affirmation is any statement made to help you validate the thoughts that you need to retrain how you think. Throughout our lives, we may start to use unhealthy affirmations, such as "I'll start on Monday" or "I'll do it later." These thoughts become natural to us, eventually creating the way that we live.

Include the healthy affirmations below in your life as often as possible to turn around the patterns of thinking that have made you want to change yourself.

We've split such affirmations into three, inclusive of the most important words of wisdom that you need in your daily life. These are all phrases that you should say to yourself as often as possible. As we read them, let them flow through your mind as if they are your own.

Write the words down to remember them further, put notes around your house with the affirmations written on them, or simply find other creative ways to incorporate them into your life. Let's start reading them now so that you can get these ideas in your head right away.

Dedication Affirmations

I am dedicated mostly to myself.

I put my health first before anything else in my life.

I am dedicated to healthy living, not any other form of life.

I am mindful of the things that I put into my body.

I make sure that I am consistently working out for my health.

I am always looking for ways to grow.

When I say that I am going to do something, I do my best to stick to it.

It feels good to be dedicated.

I am a passionate person.

Once I set my mind to something, I know what I need to do to achieve that.

I am happy when I am dedicated.

I am healthy when I am happy.

I am only focused on adding as much health as possible in my life.

I am focused on reality and how I can be happy all the time.

Everything becomes more manageable when I am dedicated.

It feels better to say 'yes' to my present self than to say 'no' to my future self.

I am always looking out for what will be the best in the future.

I am always looking for new ways to improve my health.

I am highly aware of how I can consistently boost my health.

I only add things that are good for me.

I treat myself when I need to, but I am always dedicated to being healthy so that I can quickly get back on track.

I find motivation even when I don't want to do much of anything at all.

I find ways to include better health in every aspect of my life.

I heal myself with the choices that I make.

I will always remain loyal to my health.

Self–Control Affirmations

I am patient and willing to wait for results.

I know what I need, as well as what I have to say 'no' to.

I understand what is right and wrong for me.

I am focused on practicing discipline.

I appreciate what I already have.

I do not act on impulse.

I think before I push through with a decision.

I am more durable than the biggest craving that I may feel throughout the day.

I am proud of my ability to display self-control.

I take everything in one at a time, accepting and appreciating everything that is around me.

Even the struggle is something that I am appreciative of.

I can conquer my own most prominent feelings of wanting to eat more and more.

I do not allow myself to binge eat or partake in other unhealthy patterns of eating.

I do not give into temporary urges.

I trust myself and my ability to be disciplined.

I know what I need more of and what I can do just fine with what is already there.

My temptation does not easily influence me.

I do not wait for good things to come; I take actionable steps to get them myself.

I understand that the best time to finish something is right after starting it.

I believe in my ability to make the best decisions for my health.

I don't put things off.

I do not allow procrastination in my life.

I have control over my most significant wants and desires.

I am focused only on achieving my goals.

I look out for my future self and make the best decisions with them in mind.

Healthy Living Affirmations

I can make myself feel better.

There are no outside sources that I need just to improve my health.

I do not allow anything else to make me feel unhealthy.

I know that healthy living starts in my mind.

I understand how healthy living will improve my soul.

I can feel good whenever I want.

I choose to do things that are best for my health.

I deserve to have a healthy life.

Healthy habits come naturally to me, the more I decide to let them into my body.

I am in control of the habits that I have in my life.

I am aware of the small decisions I make that can affect my health.

I understand the minor things that I can improve for the big picture of my health.

I am aware of how I need to improve my health to be able to live better.

I have a positive attitude when it comes to improving my health.

I can sacrifice certain things if it means I can start living healthier.

I am confident in my ability to know what is best for my health overall.

Each decision I make to become healthier makes me feel better.

Others see my healthy habits, and it can help encourage theirs, too.

I am excited to seek healthy habits because I know that it will help make my life better.

I always have my health at the center of my focus at the end of the day.

I am not scared of what may happen as I change my habits.

I am in control of whether I am going to live a healthy life or not.

I am dedicated to making the best decisions possible for my health.

Chapter 14: 10 Tasty And Healthy Recipes

Salmon Skewers

Preparation Time: 35 mins

Cooking Time: 30 mins

Servings: 4

Ingredients:

- ¼ c fresh spinach, chopped fine
- 1 lb. salmon cut into bite-sized pieces
- ¼ t black pepper freshly ground - ½ t pink Himalayan salt - 1 T olive oil
- 3½ oz sliced prosciutto
- 1 c full-fat mayonnaise
- Eight wooden or metal skewers

Directions:

- Heat oven to 400 degrees.
- Mix olive oil spinach salt and pepper in a 1-gallon storage bag.
- Coat salmon pieces in oil mixture by placing them in the bag.
- Place salmon on skewers.
- Wrap salmon skewers with prosciutto.
- Bake salmon for approximately 15 minutes, turning every 3 or 4 minutes.
- When prosciutto is crispy, and salmon is cooked, remove from oven.
- Serve with mayonnaise on the side.

Nutrition:

Calories: 680

Carbohydrates: 1g

Protein: 28g

Fat: 62g

Sodium: 1092 mg

Coconut Salmon with Napa Cabbage

Preparation Time: 45 mins

Cooking Time: 40 mins

Servings: 4

Ingredients:

13. 1¼ lbs. salmon - 1 T olive oil
14. ½ c unsweetened shredded coconut
15. 1 t turmeric
16. 1 t kosher salt
17. ½ t garlic powder
18. 4 T olive oil, for frying
19. 2 c. Napa cabbage
20. One stick butter
21. Salt and pepper

Directions:

7. Cut salmon into small 1-inch chunks.
8. Grind coconut to make it more likely to stay on the fish pieces. If you don't have a grinder, use a sharp knife to chop the shredded coconut as finely as possible.

9. Mix coconut, turmeric, salt, and garlic powder in a bowl. In another dish, coat salmon with one tablespoon of olive oil.

10. Take Dredge oil-coated salmon in dry ingredients. Heat 4 tablespoons of olive oil in a frying pan to medium heat.

11. Cook coconut coated salmon until crispy. It will take about one minute per side. Make sure each team gets nicely browned.

12. Remove cooked salmon from the pan and keep warm while cooking the cabbage.

13. Slice cabbage into thin strips with a knife or shred in a food processor.

14. Melt butter in pan used to cook salmon.

15. Cook cabbage until tender.

16. Season cabbage with salt and pepper.

17. Serve cabbage with salmon and enjoy it.

Nutrition:

Calories: 744

Carbohydrates: 3g

Protein: 32g

Fat: 67g

Sodium: 1457 mg

Keto Tuna Casserole

Preparation Time: 45 mins

Cooking Time: 40 mins

Servings: 4

Ingredients:

10. 4 T butter
11. 2 T olive oil
12. One medium onion, diced
13. One green bell pepper, diced
14. Five celery stalks, diced
15. 2 c baby spinach chopped fine
16. Two large cans tuna in olive oil, drained
17. 1 c mayonnaise
18. 1 ½ c freshly shredded Parmesan cheese
19. 1 t red pepper flakes
20. Salt and pepper

Directions:

- Preheat oven to 350 degrees.
- Heat butter and olive oil in a large skillet.
- Sauté onions, green bell pepper, celery, and spinach in butter/oil.
- In a bowl, mix tuna, Parmesan cheese, mayonnaise, and red pepper flake until thoroughly combined.
- Add sautéed vegetables to the tuna mixture and stir until everything is incorporated
- Pour tuna mixture into a casserole dish for baking.
- Bake in the oven for 30 minutes.
- Remove casserole from the oven when golden brown on top and bubbly.

Nutrition:

Calories: 953

Carbohydrates: 5g

Protein: 43g

Fat: 83g

Sodium: 1376 mg

Baked Fish Fillets with Vegetables in Foil

Preparation time: 10 minutes

Cooking time: 40 minutes

Servings: 3

Ingredients:

8. 1 lb. cod (or any white fish)
9. One red bell pepper, sliced
10. Six cherry tomatoes halved
11. One leek (small size, only the white part, sliced)
12. ¼ onion, sliced
13. ½ zucchini, sliced
14. One clove garlic, chopped
15. 2 tbsp olives
16. 1 oz butter
17. 2 tbsp olive oil
18. ½ lemon sliced to taste

19. Coriander leaves, to taste (optional)

20. Salt and pepper to taste

Directions:

6. Preheat oven to 400°F.

7. Slice the zucchini, leek, onion, bell pepper and lemon, cut tomatoes in half, chop the garlic.

8. Transfer all the vegetables to a baking sheet lined with foil.

9. Cut the fish into bite-sized pieces and add to the vegetables. Add salt and pepper, drizzle olive oil and add slices of butter around evenly.

10. Fold the foil and make sure you seal the joints of the foil tightly.

11. Bake for 35 – 40 minutes.

12. It can be served with aioli or any other low carb sauce of your choice.

Nutrition:

Calories: 339

Fat: 19g

Protein: 35g

Carbs: 5g

Sodium: 569 mg

Baked Salmon with Almonds and Cream Sauce

Preparation time: 10 minutes

Cooking time: 20 minutes

Servings: 2

Ingredients:

- Almond Crumbs Creamy Sauce
- 3 tbsp shaved almonds
- 2 tbsp almond milk (for thinning the sauce if necessary)
- ½ cup cream cheese
- Salt to taste
- Fish
- One salmon fillet (about ½ lb.)
- 1 tsp coconut oil
- 1 tbsp lemon zest
- 1 tsp salt

- White pepper to taste

Directions:

8. Prepare the salmon: cut the salmon in half. Mix the lemon zest, salt, and pepper and rub the mixture on the salmon. Let it cook in the refrigerator for 20 minutes so the seasonings will be absorbed. Meanwhile, preheat the oven to 300°F.

9. Heat some coconut oil on a nonstick baking dish. Fry the fish on both sides for a few minutes and make sure that the fish is sealed. Top with almond crumbs and bake in the oven for 10 to 15 minutes.

10. Take the dish out of the oven and transfer the fish to a separate plate. Set aside.

11. Place the baking dish on fire and add the cream cheese. Combine the fish cooking juices and the cheese for a more flavorful sauce.

12. Mix well until uniformed. If necessary, add some almond milk to the sauce.

13. Pour the sauce onto the fish. Best served hot.

Nutrition:

Calories 522

Fat 44g

Protein 28g

Carbs 2.4g

Sodium 1432 mg

Spring Greens Soup

Preparation time: 10 minutes

Cooking time: 30 minutes

Servings: 4

Ingredients:

- Mustard greens – Two cups, chopped
- Collard greens – Two cups, chopped
- Vegetable stock – Four cups
- Onion – 1, chopped
- Salt and ground black pepper to taste
- Coconut amino – Two Tbsp.
- Fresh ginger – 2 tsp. grated

Directions:

- Put the stock altogether into a saucepan and bring to a simmer over medium heat.
- Add ginger, coconut aminos, salt, pepper, onion, mustard, and collard greens. Stir, cover, and cook for 30 minutes. Remove from the heat.
- Blend the soup with a hand mixer.
- Serve.

Nutrition:

Calories: 35

Fat: 1g

Carb: 7g

Protein: 2g

Sodium: 64 mg

Celery Soup

Preparation time: 10 minutes

Cooking time: 30 minutes

Servings: 6

Ingredients:

- Celery – 1 bunch, chopped
- Onion – 1, chopped
- Green onion – 1 bunch, chopped
- Garlic cloves – 4, minced
- Salt and ground black pepper to taste
- Parsley – 1 fresh bunch, chopped
- Fresh mint bunches – 2, chopped
- Persian lemons – 3 dried, pricked with a fork
- Water – 2 cups
- Olive oil – 4 Tbsp.

Directions:

- Heat a saucepan with oil over medium heat.
- Add onion, garlic, and green onions. Stir and cook for 6 minutes.
- Add Persian lemons, celery, salt, pepper, water, stir, cover pan, and simmer on medium heat for 20 minutes.
- Add parsley and mint, stir, and cook for 10 minutes.
- Blend with a hand mixer and serve.

Nutrition:

Calories: 100

Fat: 9.5g

Carb: 4.4g

Protein: 1g

Sodium: 55 mg

Eggplant Stew

Preparation time: 10 minutes

Cooking time: 30 minutes

Servings: 4

Ingredients:

- Onion – 1, chopped - Garlic – 2 cloves, chopped - Fresh parsley – 1 bunch, chopped
- Salt and black pepper to taste
- Dried oregano – 1 tsp.
- Eggplants – 2, cut into chunks
- Olive oil – 2 Tbsp.
- Capers – 2 Tbsp. chopped

- Green olives – 12, pitted and sliced
- Tomatoes – 5, chopped
- Herb vinegar – 3 Tbsp.

Directions:

7. In a saucepan
8. heat oil over medium heat.
9. Add oregano, eggplant, salt, pepper, and stir-fry for 5 minutes.
10. Add parsley, onion, garlic, and stir-fry for 4 minutes.
11. Add tomatoes, vinegar, olives, capers, and stir-fry for 15 minutes.
12. Adjust seasoning and stir.
13. Serve.

Nutrition:

Calories: 280

Fat: 17.9g

Carb: 8.4g

Protein: 5.4g

Sodium: 308 mg

Asparagus Frittata

Preparation time: 10 minutes

Cooking time: 15 minutes

Servings: 4

Ingredients:

4. Onion – ¼ cup, chopped
5. A drizzle of olive oil
6. Asparagus spears – One-pound, cut into one-inch pieces
7. Salt and ground black pepper to taste
8. Eggs – four, whisked
9. Cheddar cheese – One cup, grated

Directions:

- Heat a pan with oil over medium heat.
- Add onions and stir-fry for 3 minutes.
- Add asparagus and stir-fry for 6 minutes.
- Add eggs and stir-fry for 3 minutes.
- Add salt, pepper, and sprinkle with cheese.

- Broil for 3 minutes and place it on the oven.
- Divide frittata between plates and serve.

Nutrition:

Calories: 202

Fat: 13.3g

Carb: 5.8g

Protein: 15.1g

Sodium: 106 mg

Bell Peppers Soup

Preparation time: 10 minutes

Cooking time: 15 minutes

Servings: 6

Ingredients:

7. Roasted bell peppers – 12, seeded and chopped
8. Olive oil – 2 tbsp. - Garlic – 2 cloves, minced - Vegetable stock – 30 ounces
9. Salt and black pepper to taste - Water - 6 ounces

10. Heavy cream – 2/3 cup

11. Onion – 1, chopped

12. Parmesan cheese – ¼ cup, grated

13. Celery stalks – 2, chopped

Directions:

- Heat a saucepan with oil over medium heat.
- Add onion, garlic, celery, salt, and pepper. Stir-fry for 8 minutes.
- Add water, bell peppers, stock, stir, and bring to a boil.
- Simmer for 5 minutes and cover it up and let it be.
- Remove from heat and blend with a hand mixer.
- Then adjust seasoning, and add cream. Stir and bring to a boil.
- Remove from the heat and serve on bowls.
- Sprinkle with Parmesan and serve.

Nutrition:

Calories: 155

Fat: 12g

Carb: 8.6g

Protein: 4.7g

Sodium: 90 mg

Chapter 15: Top Tips and Cautions to Stay Pescatarian

There are so many incredibly delicious foods out there that are healthy, plant-based, and keto-friendly. When Pescatarian starts to implement this diet, there are a few tricks to help you on your keto journey with minimal effort. Here are some of the best tips you should follow:

Get Your Carbs From Vegetables

While carbs are limited on the keto diet, you will need to consume a healthy amount of low-carb vegetables to supply yourself with sufficient bulk and fiber to keep your stomach full. I encourage all Pescatarian s to explore and open themselves up to new sorts of vegetables cooked in different ways. If eating vegetables raw doesn't seem tasty, try cooking the vegetables with butter or coconut oil with plenty of seasoning. Here are some low-carb vegetables you will be eating:

18. Kale
19. Collard Greens
20. Spinach
21. Swiss Chard
22. Asparagus
23. Lettuce
24. Green Beans
25. Broccoli
26. Cucumber
27. Summer Squash
28. Winter Squash
29. White Cabbage
30. Red Cabbage
31. Cauliflower
32. Bell Peppers
33. Onions
34. Mushrooms
35. Tomatoes

36. Garlic

37. Eggplants

Get Plenty Of Sleep

Establishing healthy sleep habits on a Ketogenic Pescatarian Diet will help you go to sleep faster and wake up feeling rejuvenated. Research also shows that not getting enough sleep can significantly hinder your ability to lose weight and increase your levels of stress hormones. With that said, you must prioritize sleep! If you are finding it hard to go to sleep, try taking natural sleep aids such as melatonin, which can work miracles.

Lower Your Stress

If you are suffering from chronic stress, it will interfere with your body's ability to achieve ketosis. This is because stress hormones raise your blood sugar levels, which thwarts your body's strength from burning fat for fuel. After all, there is too much glucose in your bloodstream. If you are currently going through a phase of high stress in your life, it's recommended you avoid the keto diet until you can keep the pressure at bay. You should start the keto diet when you can effectively fight off stress and commit a large portion of your time towards maintaining the state of ketosis. If you are currently dealing with stress in your life, it's still possible for you to follow the keto Pescatarian diet. All you need to do is take proper steps to reduce the amounts of stress in your life, which includes getting sufficient sleep hours, regular exercise, or practicing relaxation techniques such as deep breathing, meditation, or yoga.

Increase Your Salt Intake

A widely believed misconception is that our sodium intake should be deficient, but this is generally only an issue on high carb diets. This is because high carbohydrate diets raise your insulin levels. When insulin levels are too high, your kidney begins to retain sodium rather than extreme them. Adopting the keto diet means your insulin levels will be low, and your body excretes more salt since no carbs are dwelling in your body to spike insulin and retain sodium. Once you are in ketosis, it is recommended you add three to five grams of sodium in your diet. This will help avoid electrolyte imbalance. The best ways to ensure you get enough salt in your diet are:

Drinking homemade organic bone broth each day.

Sprinkling a little more salt onto your meals.

Adding salt to your drinking water throughout your day.

Eating salted nuts

Eating foods that naturally contain sodium, such as celery or cucumbers.

Engage In Physical Activity

Frequent exercises while on the Ketogenic Pescatarian Diet can increase your ketone levels and help you transition into ketosis much more smoothly. To achieve ketosis, your body needs to get rid of any remaining glucose in your body. Exercising uses various types of energy for fuel, including carbs, fats, and amino acids. The more you apply, the faster your body uses up its glycogen stores. Once your body completely depletes its glycogen storages, it will find alternative forms of fuel and will turn to fat for energy through the metabolic state of ketosis. Ensure to include a workout regimen that incorporates both high-intensity exercises in concurrent with low-intensity steady-state activities like walking or jogging. This will help you elevate your blood sugar levels and help your body in entering ketosis.

Keep Track Of Your Carb Macronutrients

Counting your carbohydrate intake is critical for the success of the ketogenic diet. Be sure to do your best in avoiding hidden carbs and hidden sugars in foods that appear to be keto-friendly but are not. Some examples are

Chicken wings loaded with buffalo sauce or barbecue sauce

Milk

Most fruits (berries are fine only in small quantities)

Breaded meats

Pre-packaged meals and processed foods

If you are following the Ketogenic Pescatarian Diet and the Pescatarian diet, you need to make it a habit to carefully observe the nutrition label of everything you eat until you understand the foods to avoid. The maximum amount of carbohydrates on the keto Pescatarian diet is 50 grams. When figuring out your carb count, you want to look for your daily net carb intake. To calculate your net carbs, follow the equation:

Total carbs - Fiber = Net Carbs

The rule of thumb is to have a 20 to 30 intake of net carbs per day. If you frequently exercise, you can get away with more and still maintain ketosis.

Clean Your Kitchen

You can increase your success on this diet if you only have access to healthy plant-based, keto-friendly foods in your kitchen. Many people fail on this diet due to having carb-packed meals lying around in their pantry. Cleaning out your kitchen and pantry of all unfriendly keto foods such as sugar, all-purpose flour, bread, pasta, soda, candy, rice, and legumes will force you to stick to the Pescatarian keto diet to the end. This may sound a little bit extreme, but to stay on track, you need to replace all your carb foods with keto-friendly foods.

Have Quick Meals Ready

The key to success with any diet is sticking with it. Unfortunately, mistakes are bound to happen in even our best-laid plans. There may be days where you simply can't follow the keto diet. For instance, if you are traveling and don't have time to cook, or if you are going out to eat with friends or family. For those certain occasions when you can't cook keto meals, and you need something quick to get you going, here are some easy ideas:

Keto Butter Coffee (mix one tablespoon of MCT oil and one tablespoon of butter with 1 cup of black brewed coffee)

Eat a couple of tablespoons of nut butter

Add some coconut oil or MCT oil to your morning cup of coffee or tea

Eat some dark chocolate or cheese throughout the day.

Be Mindful When Eating Out

Eating out while on the Pescatarian keto diet can be tricky. When eating out for dinner, here are a couple of ideas:

Find the restaurant website online and look at the menu ahead of time to know what is keto-compliant.

Avoid carb-packed foods such as pasta and rice dishes.

Avoid breaded and fried foods

Avoid desserts

When ordering salads, choose olive oil or vinegar rather than sugary dressings or ranch.

Tell the waiter that you are on the keto Pescatarian diet and if there are any plant-based, keto-friendly meals you can order.

The longer you follow the keto Pescatarian diet, the better you will get at recognizing keto-friendly foods. It will take some time and practice, but you will get the gist of it.

Try Meal Prepping

One of the hardest things about the keto diet is sticking to it, and meal prep makes the road easier. Think about the many times you tried diets but never have easily accessible meals ready. Meal prep can turn your refrigerator to a grab-and-go dispensator in which you can save yourself time and money, especially if you are a busy person. For some people, meal prepping can simply mean chopping your ingredients ahead of time that will be cooked later. It can also mean rationing out elements before the actual cooking process. Commonly, people prepare all the meals they plan to eat for the weak in a single day and store them inside their refrigerator.

When meal prepping, the key is always to plan. Make a list of all the meals you want to eat for the week and purchase the ingredients at the grocery accordingly beforehand. Then, you can dedicate yourself a single day to cook your meals and properly store them.

Conclusion

How long can I be on the Pescatarian ketogenic diet? Is it safe for the long-term? Many people and cultures go into ketosis and stay there for a long time without any adverse effects. Depending on your health goals, your practitioner may recommend a specific period for you to be on the ketogenic diet. Many people and cultures go into ketosis and stay there for a long time without any adverse effects.

Pescatarian ketogenic diet slims down have sincerely gone beforehand substantial in the preceding 18 months, and all matters considered. It's an unusual approach to shed those undesirable pounds brisk, but additionally, a brilliant method to get healthful and remain as such. For people who have attempted the Keto Diet are nevertheless on it; it's something aside from a consuming regimen. It's a lifestyle, a very new lifestyle. Be that as it may, much like any sizable shift in our lives, it is anything, however, a simple one, it takes a mind-boggling degree of obligation and assurance.

Bravo, But now not for all? - Although a ketogenic weight-reduction plan has been utilized to exceptionally improve individuals'satisfaction, there are some out there who do not share the more significant component's perspective. In any case, for what cause is that precisely? As a long way as we can don't forget, we were endorsed that the excellent manner of disposing of the extra weight was to stop eating the fat-filled nourishments that we're so acquainted with eating each day. So schooling individuals to consume healthful fat (The catchphrase is Healthy), you could realize why a few people would be suspicious approximately how and why you would devour progressively fat to accomplish weight loss and achieve it quickly. This concept conflicts with all that we've got ever theory nearly weight loss.

Had been created by using the liver because of starvation or if the person pursued an ingesting regimen wealthy with excessive ats and extraordinarily low carbs. Later on that 12 months, a man from the Mayo Clinic through the name of Russel Wilder named it the "Ketogenic Diet," and applied it to treat epilepsy in small children with remarkable achievement. But because of headways in medication, it became supplanted.

My Struggles Starting Keto I started Keto February twenty-eighth, 2018, I had taken a stab at the Keto Diet once before round a half yr earlier, however, was usually unable to bear the first week. The first week on Keto is the most noticeably horrible piece of the entire procedure, that is when the feared Keto Flu indicates up likewise known as the carb flu. The average response you are frame studies when changing from consuming glucose (sugar) as vitality to ingesting fats. Numerous individuals who've gone on the Keto Diet say that it seems like pulling lower back from an addictive substance. This can remain anyplace between three days to a whole week; it just kept going more than one day for my situation.

Individuals who've had the keto Flu report feeling tired, throbbing, queasy, dazed, and have lousy headaches in addition to other matters. The most critical week is ordinary, while individuals endeavoring a Keto Diet falls flat and quit. Simply do not forget this takes place to absolutely everyone from the get-go all the at the same time as, and if you can move past the initial week, the hardest component is finished. There are more than one cures you can use to help you with overcoming this unpleasant spell. Taking Electrolyte supplements, closing hydrated, consuming bone juices, eating extra meat, and getting lots of rest. Keto Flu is a deplorable occasion that jumps out at each person as the body ousts the run of the mill's regular eating regimen. You simply need to govern through.

What Does A Ketogenic Pescatarian Diet Resemble? - When the healthy individual eats a feast wealthy in carbs, their body takes the ones carbs and changes over them into glucose for fuel. Glucose is the body's essential wellspring of gas while carbs are to be had within the body, on a Keto weight loss plan there are extremely low if any in any respect carbs gobbled which powers the authority to apply different types of energy to hold the body working appropriately. This is the place healthy fat becomes probably the essential factor.

With the nonattendance of carbs, the liver takes unsaturated lipids within the organization and adjustments over them into ketone bodies.

Try no longer to devour higher than 20g of carbs every day to keep up the ordinary Ketogenic weight loss plan. I, for one, ate beneath 10g each day for an increasing number of extreme come across, but I accomplished my underlying objectives, to mention the very least. I lost 28 lbs. in a little beneath three weeks.

What Is Ketosis? When the body is energized absolutely by fat, it enters a nation called Ketosis," which is a function nation for the organization. After the whole thing of the sugars and unhealthy fat were expelled from the frame for the duration of the first couple of weeks, the structure is currently unfastened, a surprising spike in the call for wholesome fat. Ketosis has several potential benefits identified with rapid weight loss, health, or execution. In specific circumstances like sort one diabetes, inordinate ketosis can become very risky, wherein as in precise instances, mixed with discontinuous fasting may be amazingly useful for people experiencing kind two diabetes. Significant paintings are being led on this factor via Dr. Jason Fung, M.D. (Nephrologist) of the Intensive Dietary Management Program.

What I Can and Can't Eat - For another man or woman to Keto, it very well may be seeking to adhere to a low-carb diet, despite the reality that fat is the foundation of this consuming routine try not to consume all kinds of fats. Healthy fat is essential, but what are healthful fats you could inquire. Healthy fat would include grass-strengthened meats (sheep, hamburger, goat, venison), wild got fish and fish, fed red meat, and poultry. Eggs and salt-free portions of margarine can likewise be ingested. Make positive to keep away from bland vegetables, herbal products, and grains. Prepared nourishments are not the slightest bit recounted in any form or structure on the Ketogenic food plan; synthetic sugars and milk can likewise represent a severe issue.

I would like to thank you for purchasing this book and taking the time to read it. I hope that it has been helpful to you!

The Ketogenic Pescatarian diet is very beneficial for your health and stamina. Combining these two diets is one of the best you can find for your physical well-being and mental performance. Commit to it, and you will reap the benefits!

Did you like this book? Then don't forget to leave an on Amazon!

This way, other readers can get inspired too.

Do Not Go Yet, One Last Thing To Do
If you enjoyed this book or found it useful, I'd be very grateful if you'd post a short review on Amazon. Your support does make a difference, and I read all the reviews personally so I can get your feedback and make this book even better.

Thanks again for your support!

Printed in Great Britain
by Amazon